THE
BASEBALL PLAYER'S
GUIDE TO
SPORTS MEDICINE

By
PAT CROCE

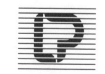
Leisure Press
Champaign, Illinois

Library of Congress Cataloging-in-Publication Data

Croce, Pat.
   Baseball player's guide to sports medicine.

   1. Baseball--Accidents and injuries.   2. Sports
medicine.   I. Title.
RC1220.B3C76 1987   617'.1027   82-83936
ISBN 0-88011-104-6

Developmental Editor: Sue Wilmoth, PhD
Production Director: Ernie Noa
Copy Editor: Kevin Neely
Proofreader: Kathy Kane
Typesetter: Theresa Bear
Text Layout: Denise Mueller
Printed By: Versa Press
Cover photo courtesy of Ray Pennacchia

ISBN: 0-88011-104-6

Printed in the United States of America

10 9 8 7 6 5 4 3 2 1

Leisure Press
A division of Human Kinetics Publishers, Inc.
Box 5076, Champaign, IL 61820

Contents

Foreword

The Baseball Player's Guide to Sports Medicine presents a whole new approach to playing, as well as coaching, our favorite sport. Developed and written by my close friend and training partner, Pat Croce, it will enable the "weekend warrior" to learn and utilize contemporary techniques for the prevention and rehabilitation of baseball's most common injuries. Pat says baseball players are very injury-prone because of the nature of the sport. Those of you who compete once or twice a week at the amateur level are even more vulnerable. This book, written by one of today's foremost authorities on sports medicine, teaches and illustrates for you proper methods of stretching and strengthening your muscles. Pat even covers emergency first-aid, something most coaches and amateur players never think about. He even offers useful expertise about nutrition and diet. Read this book and you'll become a fan of sports medicine! As a player, you owe it to yourself; as a coach, you owe it to your players. This year again I'll be using Pat's ideas in the National League. Good luck!

Mike Schmidt
Philadelphia Phillies

Preface

Baseball hasn't changed much over the years, only the players' faces. Their love for the game is no different, and their determination and dedication to the game remain the same. Skill and talent don't change. They're just borrowed, returned, and then passed on to the next generation.

But players of the past—no matter how great—can't begin to compete with the level of conditioning of today's baseball athletes. Baseball players today are healthier, more limber, and stronger. When they step onto the field, they rely on their fitness as well as their talent to win games.

Health is the newest dimension in baseball. And fans follow players' injuries and rehabilitation efforts as seriously as they memorize batting averages and win/loss records.

What's made all the difference is the rapid growth and success of a new medical specialty called sports medicine. Sports medicine uses an aggressive approach to injury treatment, not the "sit on the bench until it heals" philosophy of the past. Sports medicine experts are physicians, trainers, and therapists who love sports as much as do the players they treat. They view injured athletes not as ill patients but as healthy, vital people with an intense drive to recover. And they match that intensity with bold, innovative treatment that speeds recovery and hastens injured athletes' return to active competition.

Beyond their belief in aggressive rehabilitation, sports medicine specialists advocate injury *prevention*. To them, injuries are not unavoidable risks of the game. Athletes who condition themselves year-round are hurt less often. Simply because they can compete all season, they're the most valuable players on any baseball team. They may not be the most talented, but skill counts for little if players are benched by injuries.

What has also changed over the years is that baseball players today take an active role in their treatment and rehabilitation. No longer are they taught to follow benignly the advice and opinions of the experts who treat them. Today, specialists and athletes work together as a team, both armed with knowledge to prevent and treat injury. Physicians and trainers educate players as well as treat them because they've found that athletes who understand *why* they're being treated tend to be more committed to their rehabilitation programs. Informed players don't get lazy, they get better instead.

That's why I decided to write this book. As a physical therapist and conditioning coach, I appreciate the need for awareness on the part of the players I treat. As an athlete myself, I appreciate most what I understand best. And I do appreciate sports medicine.

You will, too, as you read through the chapters of this book. And you will finish with a far greater respect for the body you've lived in all these years. Be that body's teammate. Treat it well, satisfy its conditioning needs, and it will repay your attentiveness with 100% cooperation throughout your baseball career. Your souvenirs of the game won't be the scars of injuries suffered season after season by baseball players of the past. Conditioned and fit, you'll play longer and better than the baseball "greats" who weren't quite so healthy as you.

Pat Croce, LPT, ATC, CSCS

Acknowledgments

I wish to thank the following for their assistance in the preparation of this book: Vince Croce, who posed for demonstration pictures; Roger Schwab, of Main Line Nautilus, who provided his facility for demonstration photos; Gerald Detty, of PRO Orthopedic Devices, Inc., and Thomas Cook of Jerome Medical, who supplied their companies' athletic braces and supports; the Philadelphia Phillies management and staff, who offered their cooperation, and Janice Reeder, for her literary assistance. And I wish to express special thanks to Mike Schmidt, the Philadelphia Phillies all-star third baseman, for his invaluable insight into the world of baseball.

Chapter

1

Prevention Is the Key

You love baseball! You watch every game, memorize all the statistics, and are miserable during the off season. There may be other sports that you follow or even dabble in, but your heart always comes back to baseball. If there's a movie with a baseball story line, you'll see it. If a great baseball player appears on the *Tonight* show, you'll stay up to watch it. If there's a trivia question about the game, you know the answer.

Mainly, however, you live to *play* baseball and can't wait for the first ball to be thrown. The time you spend with your team is the highlight of the year, with every game as intense as a World Series play-off. On the field and at bat, you're a competitor— quick, aggressive, hustling. And because you are a full-fledged athlete, you're willing to risk injuries. You will do anything for your team, all for the love of baseball. After all, pain is a part of this tough game, right? You'll wear your ace bandage or your cast like a proud medal of honor, and your comrades will be proud. So what if you're sidelined by an injury? There's always the next season.

But a true baseball lover such as yourself should not be content to be knocked out of play until "next season" due to injury. That type of thinking is passé for baseball players who respect both their sport and their bodies. Of course, some bumps and bruises may be unavoidable in athletics, especially in a stand-and-sprint game like baseball. But too many injuries that sideline good players are caused by athletes' lack of physical conditioning. A slide or sprint that wouldn't faze a well-developed, regularly exercised body may wreak havoc on a player who has been plopped in front of a television since the last game of the previous season. Simply put, baseball player, you may be out of shape.

Getting in Shape

Can *athletes* be out of shape? Certainly! Being out of shape occurs all too often in both professional and amateur athletes because many players mistakenly believe that their exercise during competition provides sufficient conditioning for physical fitness. Unfortunately, however, sport participation alone cannot ensure fitness. No matter how dedicated you are when playing the game, your success on the field will be largely determined by how well you take care of and condition yourself *off* the field and during the off season. If you are blessed with an especially strong throwing arm, your natural athletic gift won't mean much if your arm is in a sling from abuse or misuse. Instead, players with less ability may take your place on the mound or in the field. Furthermore, if those players have taken the time and effort to condition on a year-round basis, they will likely replace you more and more frequently. Then, while you wither on the bench, all of your devotion to baseball and dedication to your team will not matter very much. If you are injured, you'll remain a fan instead of a participant.

The plain fact is that you cannot get in shape by playing baseball. Instead, you must get in shape to play baseball!

But many players fail to recognize the importance of getting and keeping their bodies in shape. During the late fall and early winter months, they lighten their exercise schedules or eliminate workouts from their schedules entirely. By the time the new year rolls around, they are recovering from overindulgence in holiday food and drink. Fitness becomes a mere memory from the past. Aches, pains, stiffness, and an extra 10 pounds or so sneak up on players faster than they can say "pass the popcorn, please." Finally, with news items about the approach of the spring training season, these sedentary players begin to think about resuming their beloved sport. Simultaneously, however, their muscles are deep into a winter hibernation period. But without so much as skipping a beat, many players lug their out-of-shape bodies onto the practice or—worse yet—playing field and throw themselves into rigorous play. These players are setting themselves up as prime candidates for injury.

Why? Because a body that is shocked into rigorous physical activity with little or no conditioning and preparation is statistically much more likely to be injured than one that has been regularly conditioned through exercise. Participating in baseball without physical conditioning in advance is like acting in a play with no rehearsal: There's little chance that you'll make much of an impact on the audience. Think about what would happen to a car if you failed to tune it up or add oil to the engine all winter. Eventually, after months of neglect, the car probably wouldn't start when you tried to take it for a spin the first day of spring.

The same principle holds true for that machine known as your body. It can't simply react to the words, "play ball!" after a long period of inactivity. Your body must acclimate itself to playing baseball, just like your eyes must adjust to light when you step from darkness into the sunshine.

A Solid Conditioning Program

For baseball players and their fellow athletes, preventive care begins with regular physical conditioning. Basically, conditioning involves a solid program designed to develop flexibility, endurance, and strength. As you'll see in greater detail later in this book, these three aspects of fitness are essential for baseball players who want to perform to their maximum ability and prevent sports injuries. For example, increased flexibility helps players stay loose and avoid painful pulls, such as hamstring or groin strains, when they suddenly dart to the left or right to catch a sudden pop fly. Players who have worked to increase their endurance through intense and consistent exercise (running, rowing, bicycling) are able to last through extra-inning games and avoid the painful injuries that often befall easily exhausted, out-of-shape muscles. In addition, players who build up their strength throughout the off season and into the regular season are much more able to bear up to the rigors of the game than those who rely solely on raw talent or guts. Equally important is the fact that players who have strength-trained recover from injuries more quickly than those who have not. The conditioned muscles surrounding the injured area are strong enough to support the recovering section, which allows the player to make a quick and healthy return to play.

Of course, the problems associated with any conditioning program are problems of time and commitment. A fit body requires continuous effort and lots of exercise. Even the most committed athletes admit they hate to exercise and exert all that sweat and strain. After all, exercise is hard work, and to gain any benefits you must adhere to your conditioning program year-round, not only during preseason training. That means continuing to exercise on a regular basis even after you hang your baseball cap in the closet for the winter. That means engaging in a regular indoor exercise program that can be followed regardless of weather variances to keep yourself in shape through the harsh winter months. That means adopting a sensible diet and reducing the amount of fat and cholesterol you consume. That means adopting a more healthy life style throughout the year, not only when spring has sprung.

Conditioning is essential if you want to end the baseball season as you began it—injury free. You would never consider playing your field position without a glove or trying to hit the ball when you've forgotten the bat. Yet players who would never consider competing gloveless or batless walk onto the field "fitless," suited up in a body that is ill-prepared to cope with the rigors of the game. Whether you are a Little Leaguer or a professional baseball player, conditioning should be as much a part of your game as your uniform and cleats.

Reducing Your Risks

Regardless of how sophisticated a science sports medicine has become or how quickly physicians and trainers can rehabilitate injured players, the best cure for injury is *preven-*

tion. Like betters at the race track who moan, "I should have. . ." or "If only I had . . .," baseball players might regretfully wish that they had taken conditioning more to heart when an injury relegates them to the spectators' section. Prevention-minded players are physically fit players. They not only think about the action on the field, but they also defend themselves against injuries by keeping their bodies in prime shape. They put as much effort *into* their bodies as they demand *from* them. As a result, they are seldom sidelined, offset the odds of being injured, and enjoy full seasons of play. And if by chance they are injured, these athletes are able to recuperate more quickly because their bodies are in such great shape overall.

If you love to play baseball, prove it by caring year-round for the most important of all pieces of baseball equipment—your body. Feed it well, provide it with enough sleep, and exercise and stretch it every day. If you are as aggressive and dedicated as you say you are, take on a conditioning program with as much gusto as you show on the field.

Then go play baseball! With reduced risks of being injured, you will spend far less time on the sidelines and more time playing better than ever before.

Chapter 2

Baseball's Stretching Strategy

Imagine yourself without muscles. No matter how strong your bones or how determined your resolve, you would be powerless to move, let alone play baseball. Muscles aren't just important to you as an athlete, they are vital components of your playing ability. As they contract and then extend to their full range of motion, they provide you with the mobility to swing, pitch, run, and throw. With them, you can play your best possible game. Without them, you're a spectator, one that can't even stand up to cheer!

Of course, few people ever lose their muscle mobility completely. They move freely, perform their jobs, and are capable of limited athletic activity. For many people, that's the extent of the demands they place on their muscles. Because they don't expect much from their muscles, they don't do much for their muscles. They seldom, if ever, exercise, and they fail to condition their bodies. Worst of all, they don't *stretch*.

Stretching is essential for good muscle health. Healthy muscles are flexible muscles. They're long, lean, and well-conditioned. When you stretch, you help your muscles to achieve and remain in the best possible shape. When you don't stretch, your muscles wither. They become short, squat, and inflexible. Whether or not they are athletes, people with unhealthy muscles tend to get injured. They develop bad backs, stiff shoulders, and sore calves. Whenever they expect a little extra from their muscles, those muscles just don't have it to give to them. Their poor muscles end up being sprained, strained, and torn.

As a baseball player you are particularly injury-prone. Sports such as hockey and soccer require continuous action. But baseball is filled with sudden starts, stops, lunges, and twists. In baseball you play in spurts; you're in the midst of the action, yet often inactive. No matter how much you've warmed up before the game, your muscles will cool down and tighten as you stand around waiting to bat or to field the ball. Suddenly, the ball is hit in your direction. It's your turn to play. Your mind snaps into readiness, and your body shifts into fourth gear. But your muscles resist. Cold and stiff, they're unable to respond. So you force them into action—and you get hurt.

To avoid muscle injury, baseball players must develop great baseline flexibility. That requires a stretching strategy that prepares muscles for periods of inactivity as well as for times of activity. In other words, you must develop such flexibility that even when your muscles have cooled down, they remain limber and ready to respond immediately to your playing needs.

Use the following strategy to develop your muscle flexibility. Read it carefully, and take heed of its "common sense" advice. Once you're finished, apply what you've learned to the accompanying 13 stretching exercises, which are specifically designed to benefit the three major muscle areas that baseball players most often use: shoulder to wrist (throwing), trunk (batting), and legs (running). Use the exercises before and after every practice session or game to develop a healthy, flexible team of muscles and stretch your ability to withstand injury.

Stretch daily.

Take your time; stretch *slowly.*

Repeat each exercise before moving on to the next one.

Easy does it; *relax* as you stretch.

Try not to bounce.

Concentrate on smooth, regular breathing.

Hold each position for 10–20 seconds.

Stretch Daily

Muscles do not become flexible by themselves. They need lots of attention and a daily stretching routine to satisfy all of your muscles' needs. Surprisingly, such a routine requires very little time. Just ten minutes a day should do it. Many articles have been written on the subject, and several books exist that outline complete, regular stretching programs, such as *Stretching For Athletics* by Pat Croce LPT, ATC (2nd ed., Leisure Press, New York, 1983.)

If you skip your stretching routine for one or several days, it's only fair to warn you that gravity will contract your muscles into tight, tense little clumps of atrophying tissue. By the time you begin stretching again, you will have lost some of the flexibility benefits you've worked so hard to gain.

Don't be a loser. Find a good stretching program, then stick with it at least ten minutes a day—every day.

Take Your Time—Stretch Slowly

No matter how limber your muscles are, don't underestimate their strength. Make a fist. Feel the strength? Flex your bicep. Feel the strength? Muscles are like rubber bands, flexible but tough. As you stretch them, they move with you. Contracted, they become rigid and provide solid support.

But muscles are like rubber bands in another way. Yank them too hard, and they snap. Muscles that are stretched too quickly can weaken and tear. Whenever you stretch, the momentum of your action helps carry muscles to their full range of motion. Slow, controlled momentum increases flexibility without reducing muscle strength. Sharp, uncontrolled momentum can jerk your muscles beyond their capacity to stretch.

When rubber bands break, you can simply get other rubber bands. But when muscles are injured, there are no replacements. You must wait until they heal.

To prevent injury, stretch slowly. Control your movements, don't let them control you.

Repeat Each Exercise Before Moving on to the Next One

When you first perform a stretching exercise, it's a little like sticking your toes in the water. Uncertain of the temperature, at first you are cautious and test the water. The first time you stretch, you carefully test your ability to exercise without pain. Once aware of your muscles' range of motion limitations, you can repeat the stretch comfortably. The second time, however, you stretch a little further. And that extra effort from you and from your muscles increases your flexibility.

Easy Does It—Relax as You Stretch

When you are tense, your muscles are tense, and tense muscles are hard to stretch. As you relax, your muscles loosen, which makes it easier to extend them to their full range of motion.

So before you stretch, relax.

Try Not to Bounce

Bouncing while stretching your muscles has effects very similar to stretching too quickly. The uncontrolled momentum yanks muscles and strains them beyond their stretching capacity. Whenever you bounce, you risk developing microtears in your muscle fibers. Such tears can cause so much pain that you'll avoid exercising for several days. Once you return to your stretching routine, your muscles will have lost some of their flexibility. Thus they'll be even more prone to injury; and if you continue to bounce, you'll only aggravate the problem.

Concentrate on Smooth, Regular Breathing

It's difficult to be tense when you're breathing easily because easy breathing is relaxed breathing. As you relax, your muscles relax and become more flexible. Many athletes make the mistake of holding their breath while they're holding a stretch. They tend to forget that muscles need oxygen in order to function. Without sufficient oxygen, muscles can't breathe. Muscles that are anoxic (without oxygen) quickly react by developing sharp, painful contractions known as cramps.

To avoid cramps, breathe while you stretch. To avoid tension, breathe smoothly and regularly.

Hold Each Position for 10–20 Seconds

Stretching conditions and "educates" your muscles. As you stretch, they are learning just how far they can extend themselves. Within each muscle fiber is a structure called a spindle. Like the spindle on a spinning wheel, your spindles hold your muscle fibers in the positions to which you stretch them. Because the purpose of stretching is to extend your muscles' range of motion, you must allow your muscles the chance to "learn" the new extensions and then to hold those positions on their spindles. Learning takes time, so give your muscles 10–20 seconds to re-educate themselves.

Stretch 1: Inferior Shoulder Stretch

Stand erect and place the right side of your body against a fence or backstop. Raise your right arm and grab the fence with your right hand. Slowly lean forward at the waist. Then place the left side of your body against the fence and repeat the stretch with your left arm.

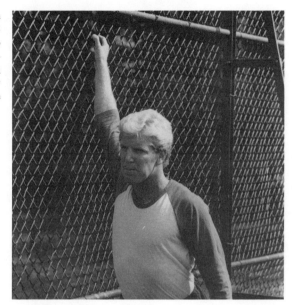

Stretch 2: Anterior Shoulder Stretch

Stand erect and place the right side of your body against a fence or backstop. Reach behind you with your right arm and grab the fence at shoulder level with your right hand. Place your left arm behind your back and grab the fence with your left hand. Look over your left shoulder and slowly rotate your trunk to the left. Then place the left side of your body against the fence, reverse arm positions, and repeat the stretch to your right.

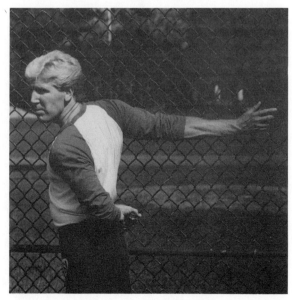

Stretch 3: Rib Stretch

Stand erect and place the right side of your body against a fence or backstop. Raise your left arm over your head and grab the fence with your left hand. Grab the fence at waist level with your right hand. Push your right hand against the fence as you slowly lean to the left. Then place the left side of your body against the fence, reverse arm positions, and lean to your right.

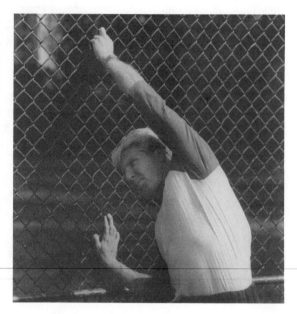

Stretch 4: Windup Stretch

Stand erect and place your back against a fence or backstop. Raise your right arm over your right shoulder and grab the fence at shoulder level with your right hand. Slowly lean forward at the waist. Repeat the stretch with your left arm.

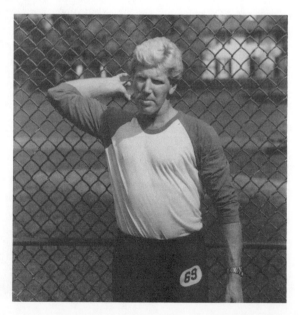

Stretch 5: Latissimus Stretch

Stand erect and face a fence or backstop. Straighten your arms, place them shoulder-width apart, and grab the fence at shoulder level. Slowly bend forward from the waist as far as you can.

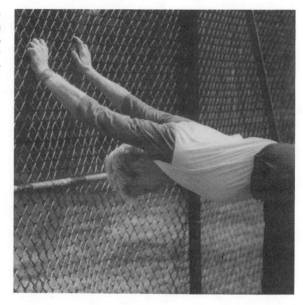

Stretch 6: Quadriceps Stretch

Stand erect. Bend your right leg and try to raise your right heel to your right buttock. Grasp your right ankle with your right hand and slowly pull your right leg toward your head. Then stretch your left leg. If necessary, hold onto a fence or backstop for support.

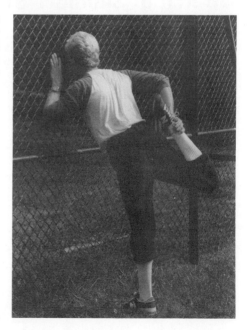

Stretch 7: Calf Stretch

Stand erect and face a fence or backstop. Straighten your legs and place your heels flat on the ground. Grab the fence for support and then slowly lean forward from your hips.

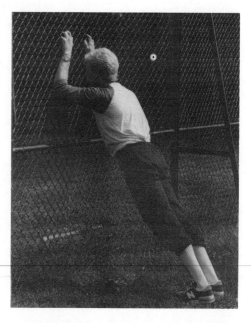

Stretch 8: Shoulder Stretch

Grab a baseball bat at both ends. Straighten your arms. Slowly lift the bat over your head and as far behind you as you can stretch without bending your elbows.

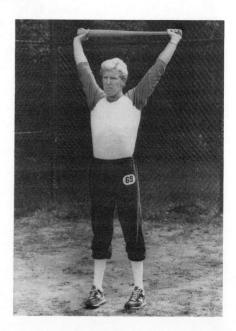

Stretch 9: Rotation Stretch

Grab a baseball bat at both ends and rest it behind your head on your shoulders. Look over your right shoulder as you slowly twist your trunk to the right. Then stretch to your left.

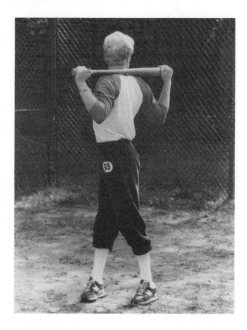

Stretch 10: Trunk Stretch

Grab a baseball bat at both ends and rest it behind your head on your shoulders. Slowly bend to your right. Then bend to your left.

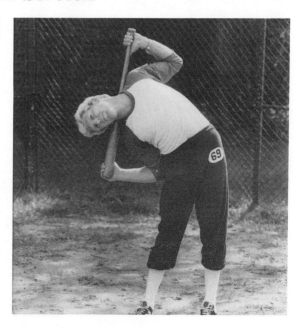

Stretch 11: Windmill Stretch

Grab a baseball bat at both ends and rest it behind your head on your shoulders. Bend forward at the waist and try to touch your left elbow to your right knee. Then twist to your left and try to touch your right elbow to your left knee.

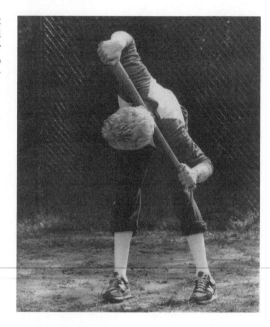

Stretch 12: Hamstrings Stretch

Grab a baseball bat at both ends. Straighten your legs and slowly bend forward. Try to touch the bat to the ground.

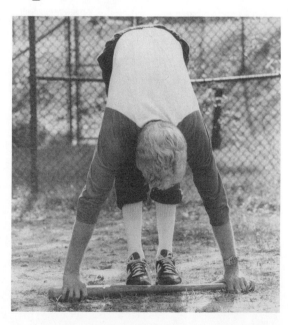

Stretch 13: Adductors Stretch

Grab a baseball bat at both ends and stand erect with your feet spread wide apart. Place your right heel firmly on the ground and then slowly bend your right leg. Keep your left leg straight and point the toes of your left food upward. Rest the bat on the ground in front of you for support. Then stand erect, reverse leg positions, and repeat the stretch.

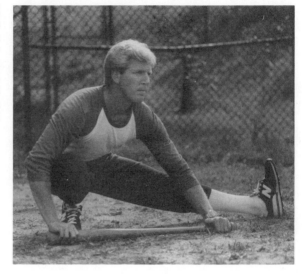

Chapter

3

Conditioning the Throwing Arm

Every player position in baseball requires an athlete with a good throwing arm. Although the pitcher is the kingpin when it comes to throwing, catchers and fielders also must be capable of throwing the ball well. Regardless of your batting talent or catching skill, you can't play baseball if you cannot throw. Throwing is vitally important to the success of a winning team.

With so much success riding on your throwing ability, it's important to both you and your team that you keep your arm healthy. Good arm health is no different than good body health. It begins with year-round conditioning and with your commitment to maintain a high level of fitness. All the throwing talent in the world won't keep you fit and playing. Conditioning takes effort and sweat, and no amount of talent can exempt any athlete from the need for regular conditioning.

The four-part conditioning program you'll find in this chapter is designed for prevention as well as rehabilitation. Simply put, what works when you're healthy will work when you're hurt—just like Vitamin C.

Four-Part Conditioning Program

   I. Stretching Routine
  II. General Arm Strengthening Routine
 III. Rotator Cuff Strengthening Routine
 IV. Throwing Routine

Part I: Stretching Routine

Your best bet for an excellent stretching program can be found in the "Baseball's Stretching Strategy" presented in chapter 2. Of the 13 stretches, six are especially designed to increase the flexibility of your arms (Stretches #1, #2, #3, #4, #5, and #8). Performing all 13 stretches before and after every game and practice session will satisfy the throwing arm's flexibility needs for most players.

Pitchers, however, throw so often, deliver with so much force, and place their throwing arms in such contorted positions that they require extra stretching to withstand the incredible stresses. Like their team members, pitchers should stretch before and after every game and practice session, whether they're pitching or sitting in the bullpen. But pitchers should also stretch their pitching arms spontaneously—wherever and whenever they can. There is no danger of too much stretching, especially when you consider that too little stretching can ruin a promising pitching career.

Players who injure their throwing arms must be as committed to stretching as they were prior to getting hurt. Injuries do *not* mean a vacation from stretching. Hurt players should perform their arm stretching exercises twice a day or more, depending on the advice of their physicians and athletic trainers. Without regular stretching, throwing arm muscles become short, squat, and inflexible and can be easily reinjured when play is resumed. Stretching when you're injured may hurt, but it will hurt a lot more if you can't compete because you fail to stretch.

Part II: General Arm Strengthening Routine

Strengthening your throwing arm is as important to your conditioning program as maintaining your muscle flexibility. Strong, flexible players are the best possible players, and they tend to get injured much less frequently. The primary reason for this reduction in injuries is that players who condition themselves for both strength and flexibility are building a balance between muscle bulk and muscle leanness. Heavier, thicker muscles produce power that is needed to give speed and distance to pitched or thrown balls. Long, lean muscles extend the throwing arm to its full range of motion so that the arm's strength cannot yank its muscles beyond any limits where injuries may occur due to lack of exercise.

Muscles that are too bulky reduce upper body agility, somewhat similar to the effect of wearing layers upon layers of winter clothing while trying to throw a ball. But muscles that are too long and lean don't generate power. Pitching the ball might be easy, but it'll go nowhere slowly.

The key is to develop a balance between muscle strength and muscle flexibility. You need to stretch and strengthen your throwing arm with equal dedication—whether your're healthy or injured—for both prevention and rehabilitation.

Before you begin the "General Arm Strengthening Routine," pay close attention to the following strength training rules. As with stretching, there's a right way and a wrong way to train for muscle strength.

Here's the right way:

Strength Training Rules

- Perform each strength exercise slowly and smoothly.
- Concentrate on proper form—no cheating!
- Avoid twisting your body or shifting your weight as you lift the weights.
- Breathe properly as you train. Take a deep breath before you lift and then exhale through your mouth during the contraction.
- For each exercise, select a weight that allows you to perform between eight and twelve repetitions.
- Continue each exercise until you can no longer do any repetitions. But as soon as you are able to perform 12 repetitions, you can increase the resistance during the next workout by five pounds.
- Perform 1 to 3 sets of each exercise.
- For best results, perform the exercises in the order described.
- Strength train on alternate days, no more than three times a week.
- Record your strength training progress in the "Conditioning the Throwing Arm Diary" on page 35.

The following exercises have been tailored to meet your physical needs as a baseball player. Each set of two exercises strengthens specific muscles through the use of Nautilus equipment and dumbbell weights. Don't worry about getting too "muscle bound." You'll build strength, but not bulk. And if you continue stretching as you strength train, you'll build balance, too. And that is what you want.

Exercises for General Arm Strengthening

MUSCLES AFFECTED	NAUTILUS MACHINE	DUMBBELLS
Pectorals	#1 Double Chest Machine	#1 Butterflies
Rhomboids	#2 Rowing Machine	#2 Reverse Butterflies
Latissimus Dorsi	#3 Super Pullover Machine	#3 Shoulder Extensions
Deltoids	#4 Lateral Raise Machine	#4 Lateral Raises
Triceps	#5 Multi-Tricep Machine	#5 Elbow Extensions
Biceps	#6 Multi-Bicep Machine	#6 Elbow Curls
Wrist Extensors	#7 Multi-Exercise Machine	#7 Wrist Extensions
Wrist Flexors	#8 Multi-Exercise Machine	#8 Wrist Curls

Nautilus Exercise #1

Double Chest Machine (Arm Cross)

Adjust the seat of the Nautilus machine so that your shoulder joints are directly under the axes of the overhead cams. Fasten your seat belt. Place your forearms behind and firmly against the movement arm pads. Grasp the handles and then slowly begin pushing with your forearms. Try to bring your elbows together in front of your chest.

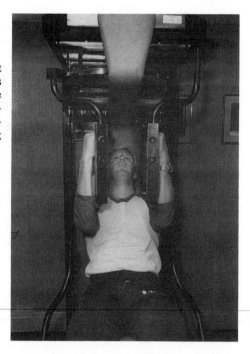

Dumbbell Exercise #1

Butterflies

Lie supine on a bench and grasp a dumbbell in each hand. Slightly bend your elbows and place them at shoulder level. Slowly push the dumbbells upward and together over your chest.

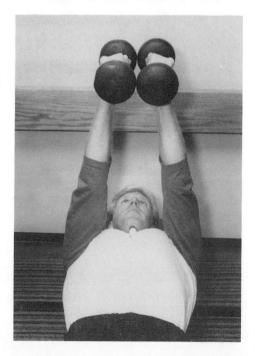

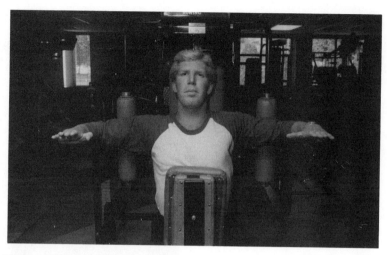

Nautilus Exercise #2

Rowing Machine

Sit down and place your back flat against the back of the seat. Place your arms between the pads. Bend your elbows and then cross your arms in front of you. Slowly pull your arms backward as far as possible. Be sure to keep your elbows bent and at shoulder level.

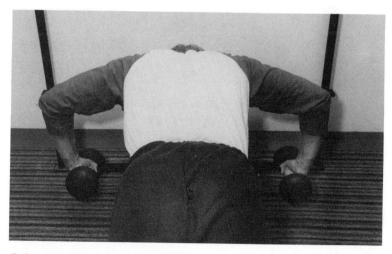

Dumbbell Exercise #2

Reverse Butterflies

Lie prone on a bench and grasp a dumbbell in each hand. Slightly bend your elbows and place the elbows at shoulder level. Slowly pull your arms upward as far as possible.

Nautilus Exercise #3

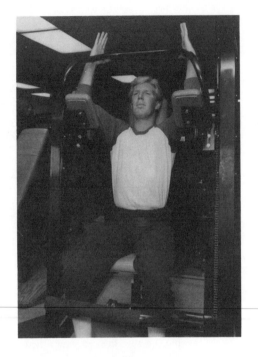

Super Pullover Machine

Adjust the seat of the Nautilus machine so that your shoulder joints align with the axes of the cams. Fasten your seat belt. Push on the foot pedal until the machines's elbow pads are at eye level. Place your elbows on the pads and rest your hands on the crossbar. Begin the exercise with your arms placed as far as possible behind your head. Slowly push with your elbows until the bar touches your body's midsection.

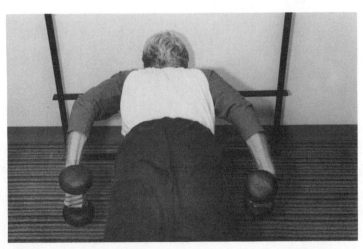

Dumbbell Exercise #3

Shoulder Extensions

Lie prone on a bench and grasp a dumbbell in each hand. Slightly bend your elbows and place your arms directly below your shoulders. Slowly pull your arms backward as far as possible. Be sure to keep your elbows bent.

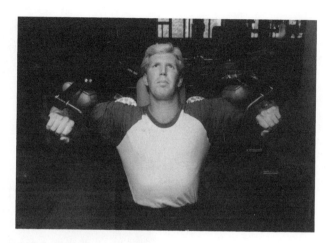

Nautilus Exercise #4

Lateral Raise Machine

Adjust the seat of the Nautilus machine so that, with your arms raised, your shoulder joints align with the axes of the cams. Fasten your seat belt. Place your forearms firmly against the pads and grasp the handles. Slowly push with your forearms until your elbows are parallel to the floor.

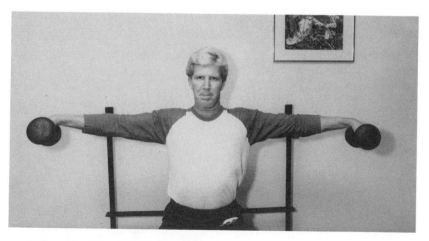

Dumbbell Exercise #4

Lateral Raises

Sit on a bench and grasp a dumbbell in each hand. Slightly bend your elbows and place your fore-arms against the sides of your body. Slowly lift your arms upward and then outward until your forearms are parallel to the floor. Be sure to keep your elbows bent throughout the exercise.

Nautilus Exercise #5

Multi-Tricep Machine

Adjust the seat of the Nautilus machine so that your shoulders are positioned slightly lower than your elbows. Place your elbows on the pads in alignment with the axes of the cams. Place your hands on the movement arm pads and bend your elbows as much as possible. Then straighten your elbows by slowly pushing with your hands.

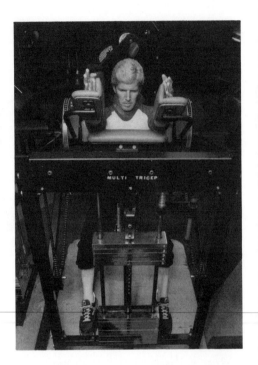

Dumbbell Exercise #5

Elbow Extensions

Lie supine on a bench and grasp a dumbbell with your right hand. Bend your right elbow as much as you can and position the elbow directly over your right shoulder. For additional support, place your left hand beneath your right elbow. Straighten your right elbow by slowly pushing upward with your right hand. Then reverse arm positions and repeat the exercise.

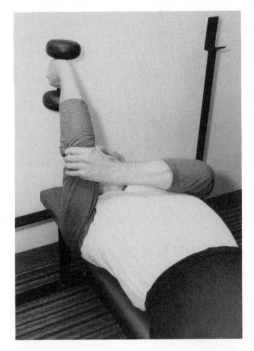

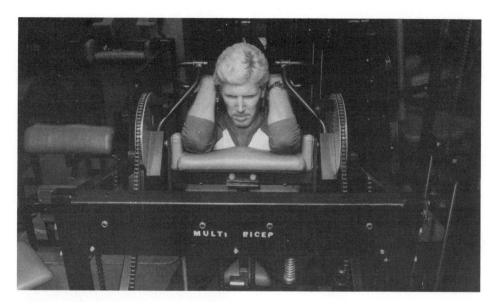

Nautilus Exercise #6

Multi-Bicep Machine

Adjust the seat of the Nautilus machine so that your shoulders are positioned slightly lower than your elbows. Place your elbows on the pads in alignment with the axes of the cams. Grasp the handles in a "palms-up" position. Begin the exercise by extending your elbows. Then slowly pull backward with your hands as far as possible.

Dumbbell Exercise #6

Elbow Curls

Sit on a bench and grasp a dumbbell in your right hand. Begin the exercise by extending your right elbow and then resting the elbow against your inner thigh. For additional support, grasp your right thigh with your left hand in a position directly behind your right elbow. Slowly pull upward as far as possible with your right hand. Then reverse arm positions and repeat the exercise.

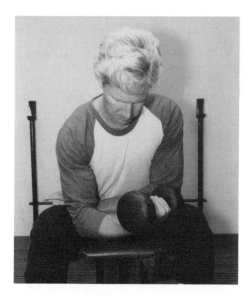

Nautilus Exercise #7

Multi-Exercise Machine (Wrist Extension)
Sit in a chair and face the Nautilus machine. Place your toes underneath the first step. Bend your elbows at a 90° angle, then rest your forearms on your thighs. Grasp the machine's handles in a "palms-down" position. Slowly pull upward as far as possible with your hands without removing your forearms from your thighs.

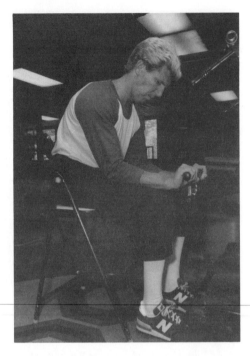

Dumbbell Exercise #7

Wrist Extensions
Sit in a chair and grasp a dumbbell in each hand. Bend your elbows at a 90° angle, then rest your forearms on your thighs. Rest your wrists over the ends of your knees and place your hands in a "palms-down" position. Slowly pull upward with your hands as far as possible without removing your forearms from your thighs.

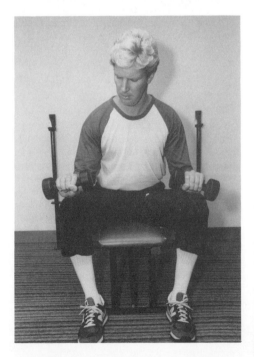

Nautilus Exercise #8

Multi-Exercise Machine (Wrist Curls)
Sit in a chair and face the Nautilus machine. Place your toes underneath the first step. Bend your elbows at a 90°angle, then rest your forearms on your thighs. Grasp the machine's handles in a "palms-up" position. Slowly pull upward as far as possible with your hands without removing your forearms from your thighs.

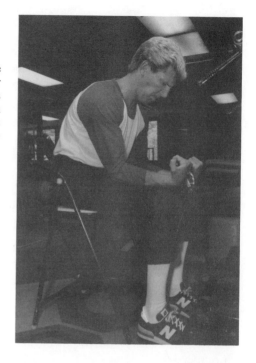

Dumbbell Exercise #8

Wrist Curls
Sit in a chair and grasp a dumbbell in each hand. Bend your elbows at a 90°angle, then rest your forearms on your thighs. Rest your wrists over the ends of your knees and place your hands in a "palms-up" position. Slowly pull upward as far as possible with your hands without removing your forearms from your thighs.

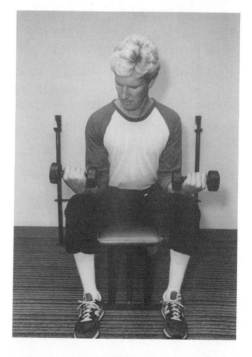

Part III: Rotator Cuff Strengthening Routine

Once you have developed adequate strength and flexibility for your entire throwing arm, you should concentrate your efforts on strengthening the rotator cuff muscles, which are injured all too often by baseball players, especially pitchers.

Your rotator cuffs are composed of muscles and tendons that encircle and support your shoulder joints. Whenever you raise your throwing arm over your head to throw the ball, you are relying on the strength and flexibility of your rotator cuff muscles from the initiation of the throw to the follow-through.

Many pitches and throws in baseball involve overhand motions, so it's important for the rotator cuff muscles to be in great shape. The arm stretching exercises in chapter 2 will help to make these muscles limber. As for strength, you'll need extra conditioning to generate the power you need for the throw.

Strength training is especially important for baseball players with rotator cuff injuries. Most such conditions are caused when rotator cuff tendons tear and become inflamed as a result of repeated rubbing against the shoulder blade. The resulting injury is *tendonitis,* and the treatment for such an injury involves reducing the pain and swelling. While the tendons are being treated, however, the muscles are weakening from disuse. Far too many players return to competition with cured tendonitis but with weakened muscles, reduced power, and a strength/flexibility imbalance that results in reinjury.

The solution to this dilemma is to treat the tendonitis *and* strengthen the muscles. Then—and only then—should the player return to active play. Sports medicine treatments were never meant to induce one injury while treating another.

The following three exercises for rotator cuff strengthening are beneficial to both healthy and injured athletes. Injured players, however, should check with their physician or athletic trainer before starting this routine.

As with the general arm-strengthening exercises, follow the strength training rules for best results.

Exercises for Rotator Cuff Strengthening

#1	Internal Rotation Curls	(Use barbell)
#2	External Rotation Curls	(Use barbell)
#3	Throwing Curls	(Use dumbbell)

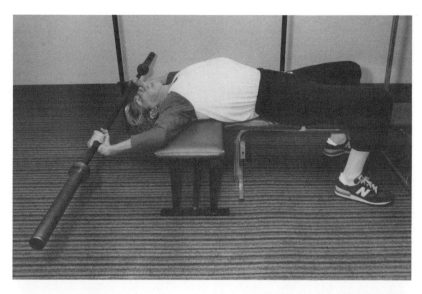

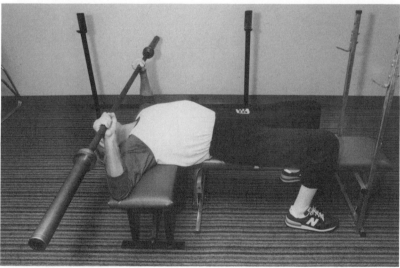

Rotator Cuff Exercise #1

Internal Rotation Curls

Lie supine on a T-shaped bench. (If necessary, place two exercise benches perpendicular to each other so that they form a "T.") Rest your head over the edge of the bench. With your elbows bent at a 90°angle, grasp a barbell with both hands. Rest your elbows on the bench's edge at shoulder level and place the barbell as far as possible behind your head. Slowly pull your arms forward and upward until your forearms are perpendicular to the floor. Be sure to keep your elbows bent, at shoulder level, and on the bench.

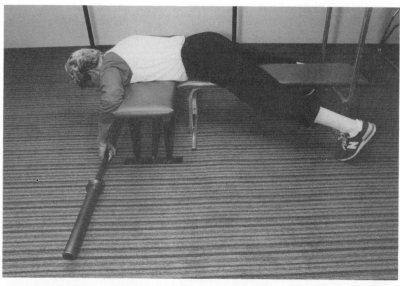

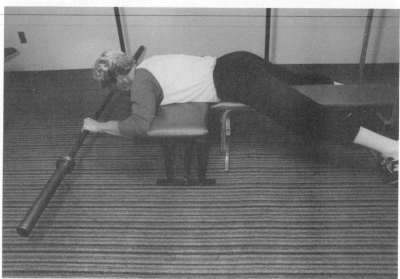

Rotator Cuff Exercise #2

External Rotation Curls

Lie prone on a T-shaped bench. (If necessary, place two exercise benches perpendicular to each other so that they form a "T.") Place your chin over the edge of the bench. With your elbows bent at a 90°angle, grasp a barbell with both hands. Place your forearms against the edges of the bench and perpendicular to the floor with your elbows at shoulder level. Slowly pull your arms upward until they are parallel to the floor.

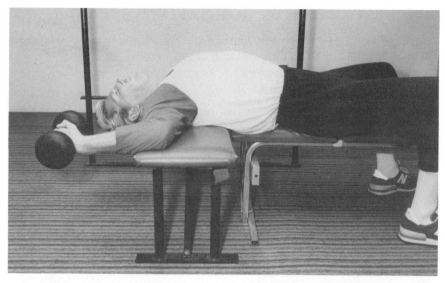

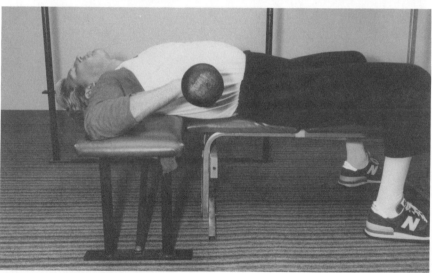

Rotator Cuff Exercise #3

Throwing Curls

Lie supine on a T-shaped bench. (If necessary, place two exercise benches perpendicular to each other so that they form a "T.") Place your head over the edge of the bench. With your elbow bent at a 90°angle, grasp a dumbbell with your throwing arm. Rest your elbow on the bench's edge at shoulder level and place the dumbbell as far as possible behind your head. Slowly push your arm forward and then pull it backward, as far as possible in both directions. Keep your elbow on the bench.

Part IV: Throwing Routine

No conditioning routine will benefit your throwing arm better than the act of throwing itself. Beyond its necessity in the game of baseball, throwing is a great training tool. It prepares stretched, strengthened muscles for the upcoming season or for re-entry into competition following an injury.

The accompanying 3-week throwing routine should be undertaken only after your throwing arm is strong and flexible enough to withstand the rigors of the throwing or pitching motion. It is a six-phase program that slowly and effectively works your arm muscles into peak condition.

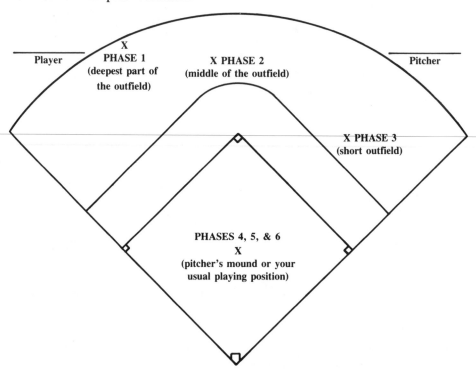

Phase 1.   Make long, easy throws from the deepest part of the outfield to home plate. Continue to throw for 20 minutes on 2 consecutive days. Then refrain from throwing for 2 days.

Phase 2.   Move to the middle of the outfield. Concentrate on stronger throws, allowing the ball to bounce four or five times before reaching home plate. Continue Phase 2 for 20 minutes on 2 consecutive days. Then refrain from throwing for 1 day.

Phase 3.   Move to the short outfield and use strong, sharp throws to reach home plate. The ball should bounce only once in the process. Continue to throw for 20 minutes on 2 consecutive days. Then refrain from throwing for 1 day.

Phase 4.   Return to the pitcher's mound or to your regular playing position. Throw to all bases at half speed without allowing the ball to bounce. Continue to throw for 15 minutes, then refrain from throwing for 1 day.

Phase 5.   Follow the directions in Phase 4. At the end of 15 minutes, throw for 5 minutes at three-quarter speed. Refrain from throwing for 1 day. Then repeat Phase 5 and refrain again on the following day.

Phase 6.   Throw to all bases from your regular position for 15 minutes at three-quarter speed. Concentrate on accuracy and proper throwing rhythm. Refrain from throwing for 1 day. Then repeat Phase 6 and refrain again on the following day.

Now that you've completed all six phases, you're ready for practice sessions and for competition. Good luck!

A Six-Phase Throwing Routine
Your Three-Week Chart

WEEK #1	PHASE	DURATION	INTENSITY	LOCATION
Monday	1	20 min.	long & easy	deep outfield
Tuesday	1	20 min.	long & easy	deep outfield
Wednesday	Rest	-----	-----	-----
Thursday	Rest	-----	-----	-----
Friday	2	20 min.	long & strong	middle outfield
Saturday	2	20 min.	long & strong	middle outfield
Sunday	Rest	-----	-----	-----
WEEK #2				
Monday	3	20 min.	strong & sharp	short outfield
Tuesday	3	20 min.	strong & sharp	short outfield
Wednesday	Rest	-----	-----	-----
Thursday	4	15 min.	1/2 speed	playing position
Friday	Rest	-----	-----	-----
Saturday	5	20 min.	1/2 & 3/4 speeds	playing position
Sunday	Rest	-----	-----	-----
WEEK #3				
Monday	5	20 min.	1/2 & 3/4 speeds	playing position
Tuesday	Rest	-----	-----	-----
Wednesday	6	15 min.	3/4 speed	playing position
Thursday	Rest	-----	-----	-----
Friday	6	15 min.	3/4 speed	playing position
Saturday	Rest	-----	-----	-----
Sunday	Practice	-----	full speed	-----

The following diary will help you to record your progress throughout the four-part conditioning program. The diary is set up for three weeks, but your program is year-round. Make additional copies of your diary as you continue, and make your fitness statistics as important to your baseball career as your batting average and fielding record.

As you can see, stretching should be done every day. The need to stretch never stops if you want to keep limber. Strengthen your muscles three times a week, with time between each session so that your muscle fibers can repair and rebuild themselves after the rigors of weight training. Throwing sessions should be conducted four times weekly, with periodic days of rest.

Conditioning the Throwing Arm
Your Three-Week Diary

WEEK #1	Stretching	Strengthening	Throwing	Phase
Monday	X	X	X	(1)
Tuesday	X		X	(1)
Wednesday	X	X		( )
Thursday	X			( )
Friday	X	X	X	(2)
Saturday	X		X	(2)
Sunday	X			( )
WEEK #2				
Monday	X	X	X	(3)
Tuesday	X		X	(3)
Wednesday	X	X		( )
Thursday	X		X	(4)
Friday	X	X		( )
Saturday	X		X	(5)
Sunday	X			( )
WEEK #3				
Monday	X	X	X	(5)
Tuesday	X			( )
Wednesday	X	X	X	(6)
Thursday	X			( )
Friday	X	X	X	(6)
Saturday	X			( )
Sunday	X		X	(6)

Conditioning the Throwing Arm
Your Three-Week Diary

WEEK #1	Stretching	Strengthening	Throwing	Phase
Monday	_____	_____	_____	( )
Tuesday	_____	_____	_____	( )
Wednesday	_____	_____	_____	( )
Thursday	_____	_____	_____	( )
Friday	_____	_____	_____	( )
Saturday	_____	_____	_____	( )
Sunday	_____	_____	_____	( )
WEEK #2				
Monday	_____	_____	_____	( )
Tuesday	_____	_____	_____	( )
Wednesday	_____	_____	_____	( )
Thursday	_____	_____	_____	( )
Friday	_____	_____	_____	( )
Saturday	_____	_____	_____	( )
Sunday	_____	_____	_____	( )
WEEK #3				
Monday	_____	_____	_____	( )
Tuesday	_____	_____	_____	( )
Wednesday	_____	_____	_____	( )
Thursday	_____	_____	_____	( )
Friday	_____	_____	_____	( )
Saturday	_____	_____	_____	( )
Sunday	_____	_____	_____	( )

Chapter

4

Emergency First Aid

Baseball injuries cannot be ignored. Once they occur, they must be treated—not after the game, not several days later, but *immediately*. Initial treatment is just as important as any specialized care administered later because when treatment begins, healing begins, and the game can resume with all players participating.

Nowadays many teams have trainers and/or physicians who treat injured athletes. But you as a player can't always count on the presence of such medical experts at practices or games. Your team may not have doctors or trainers. So when injuries occur, any immediate first aid must be rendered by the coach or by the players themselves.

The information in this chapter will not make you a medical expert, so don't fool yourself into thinking that you can treat any injury. What chapter 4 will provide are some sound tips for handling injured teammates. The material presented in chapter 4 is basic, but mastering it will enable you to give injured players a valuable head start to recovery.

Evaluation of an Unconscious Player

Baseball may not be a contact sport, but occasionally a player is knocked unconscious during a game. The causes are varied—getting hit by a beanball, diving head first into a base, fainting from heat exhaustion on a hot summer day.

Whatever the cause, unconscious players must be treated very carefully. Without their personal input about the extent of their injuries, any first aid efforts are based somewhat on guesswork.

Your first objective in administering first aid to an unconscious player is to ensure that the athlete is breathing and has a pulse. Cardiopulmonary resuscitation (CPR) instructors call this the "ABCs" of emergency rescue. First, establish an airway, then begin rescue breathing if necessary. Next check for blood circulation by finding a pulse. In the absence of breathing and a pulse, begin CPR.

If you're not CPR-certified, you won't be able to perform the previous three steps. These steps are highly effective, but you need specialized training to administer them. CPR courses are offered regularly throughout the United States and in other countries. The classes are inexpensive and are usually available both days and evenings for your convenience. If you haven't received CPR training, don't wait for an actual emergency to regret your lack of knowledge. Sign up soon and learn how to administer CPR.

Let's assume that you are CPR-certified. Check the athlete's breathing and pulse, then get as many facts as you can about the cause of unconsciousness. Ask teammates and spectators if they witnessed the accident and try to determine how it occurred.

Once you've gathered information, begin to look for injuries. Start with the player's head. Is bleeding evident? Is fluid draining from the eyes, ears, nose, or mouth? Look and feel for bumps, lacerations, or deformities that may indicate a possible concussion or skull fracture. Next, slowly move down the player's body and check the trunk, pelvis, and each limb for swelling, bleeding or deformities.

If at all possible, try to arouse the unconscious athlete. Wave ammonia capsules under the nose and tap the player lightly on the face. Do not shake the person, however. If there is a back or neck injury, any movement can aggravate the problem.

Whatever your findings, do not move the unconscious player until physicians, athletic trainers, or emergency personnel have arrived to supervise transportation off the field. Report your findings to them and let them make all further decisions regarding the athlete's care. Neither they nor you should be too hasty to move the athlete because the game is being held up to administer on-the-field treatment. The safety of an injured player is far more important than continuing the game.

If an emergency crew has arrived with an ambulance, they will transport the injured athlete. In the absence of an ambulance and crew, teammates should transport the injured player with care. Treat such a transport as if the player had a fractured spine. You just can't be too cautious. Five transporters are required. One person at the player's head supports the head and neck; three people, all on the same side of the injured player, support the trunk, pelvis and legs; and one person carefully slides a stretcher or other sturdy support underneath the unconscious athlete. Immobilize the player as much as possible and then slowly carry the athlete off the field.

Remember, treating an unconscious athlete is like waiting for a pitch. You don't swing until you see what's being thrown. Similarly, do not make any hasty first aid decisions without the facts and knowledge necessary to administer treatment safely and effectively.

Evaluating an Injury

When it comes to making an initial evaluation of an injury, trust your senses: *look, listen, and feel.*

Look. A careful visual examination of an injured player will allow you to detect swelling, bleeding, skin discoloration, and obvious deformities. Limb deformities are sure signs of fractures and/or dislocations.

Listen. If the injured athlete is conscious, he or she is your best source of information in locating the injury and determining its seriousness. Ask the athlete how the injury occurred and whether he or she heard any unusual sounds at the time of the injury. A snap, crackle, or pop may indicate that a bone was broken or a ligament torn.

Feel. Feeling or "palpating" an injured area can reveal both the nature and the severity of a wound. Be very careful as you feel. Don't aggravate the injury with unnecessary pressure.

Emergency Splinting

Often your initial evaluation of an injury cannot differentiate between dislocations, sprains, and fractures. The symptoms of these three types of injuries are similar, and accurate diagnosis requires examination by a physician.

If you are not such a specialist, treat these injuries as if they were fractures. It is much better to be overly cautious than overly careless. Immediate treatment of a fracture involves splinting, the application of a rigid support to immobilize the injured limb. Properly applied, splints lessen an injured athlete's pain, minimize swelling, and reduce the danger that a fractured bone will break through the skin, thereby increasing the risk of infection.

Splinting Guidelines

- Never attempt to reduce or straighten a dislocation or fracture. Splint the injured limb as is and let the physicians take care of the rest.
- Splint firmly for support, but avoid impeding blood circulation.
- Make the splint long enough to immobilize the limb above and below the injury site. If the splints available are too short, then make two splints, one above and one below the injury.

Many professional and amateur baseball teams include commercially prepared splints as part of their first aid equipment. You can select from prepadded board splints, molded aluminum splints, air inflatable splints, and long and short backboards.

But splints do not have to be commercially sold products. Any item can be used as a splint as long as it can immobilize a fracture, dislocation, or sprain. Tongue depressors, for instance, make excellent finger splints. Injured arms and legs can be supported by baseball bats, canes, short lengths of wood, or tightly rolled newspapers. Even blankets make effective splints. Pillows, too, are great for immobilizing ankles and feet.

To immobilize an athlete with a suspected back injury, use doors, ladders, or wide planks of wood. Unconscious players also should be handled in such a fashion. Until they are thoroughly examined off the field by qualified personnel, these athletes must be treated with the utmost care.

The following four illustrations provide helpful hints for splinting shoulders, elbows, fingers, ankles, and feet. Practice these techniques in nonemergency conditions until you are adept at applying the splints. Injured athletes will gain no reassurance from your struggling through the directions as they lie on the field in pain.

Emergency Splinting

Sling and swathe for shoulder injuries.

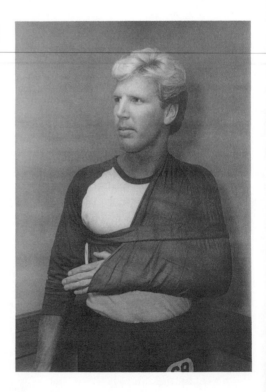

Emergency Splinting

Padded board splint and ace bandage for elbow injuries.

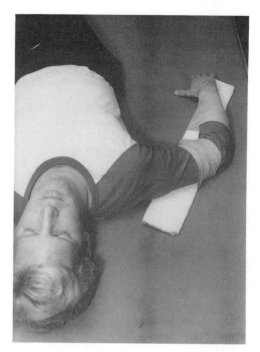

Emergency Splinting

Tongue depressor splint for finger injuries.

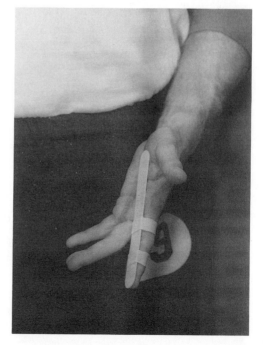

Emergency Splinting

Pillow splint for ankle/foot injuries.

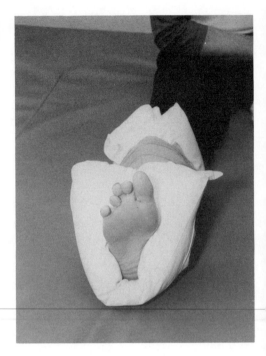

The RICE Principle

Whether you have pulled a muscle, sprained a ligament, dislocated a joint, or broken a bone, the immediate treatment for these and almost all injuries is RICE, an acronym meaning *rest, ice, compression,* and *elevation.*

R*est.* Once you have been injured, continuing to play will only increase the severity of the wound. Stop playing immediately and use your injured limb as little as possible. If you sprain your ankle, for example, you'll have to use crutches so that your ankle does not bear any weight.

I*ce.* Cold constricts ruptured blood vessels and thus reduces bleeding and swelling. Cold also decreases inflammation, muscle spasm, and pain. Any form of cold application such as an ice bag, cold bath, or frozen gel pack will do the trick.

To apply cold, first place a towel over the affected area. Then place your cold application over the towel. Don't apply the ice directly to the skin because this will cause an uncomfortable burning sensation.

Apply ice to your injury every 4 hours for 10–20 minutes. Avoid icing for more than 30 minutes. Continuous icing for a half hour or more can dilate your blood vessels, resulting in increased blood flow to the injury, which is just the opposite of what you want.

Compression. Applying an elastic ace wrap bandage to the injury reduces swelling by preventing the accumulation of blood and lymph. Place the bandage directly over the cold application. Be careful not to wrap the bandage too tightly. After you have iced the injury for 10-20 minutes, unwrap the bandage, remove the cold application, and then rewrap the bandage.

Avoid wearing a compression bandage when you sleep. Unwrap the bandage before you go to bed, then rewrap it when you get up.

Elevation. Raising the affected area above the level of your heart permits gravity to prevent excess fluid from accumulating. During the night, for instance, place a pillow under your injured limb. To elevate a leg, you can also place the foot of your bed upon blocks.

Too many players do nothing for injuries until several days after they have been hurt. By that time, the swelling, inflammation, and pain is so unbearable that they are forced to seek treatment. Be sensible about your injuries. When you have been hurt, the first 48 hours are critical. The more immediate the treatment, the faster the injury will heal. Don't be a hero by trying to ignore an injury and letting it go untreated. Seek appropriate treatment immediately to allow quick recovery, and be a hero when you play.

Chapter
5

Care of the
Common
Conditions

In learning about different kinds of injuries, you can be easily overwhelmed by the seemingly endless types of injuries that baseball players can incur.

Don't get frustrated. The injuries you encounter may change somewhat from one limb or muscle to another, but almost every injury can be categorized into one of seven common conditions.

Learning about injuries is a little like learning how to play baseball. You begin with the basics and then advance to more complex variations. In this chapter, you'll find the definitions, causes, and treatments for the seven common injury conditions, including abrasions, blisters, contusions, lacerations, ligament sprains, muscle strains, and tendonitis. An eighth common injury condition, the fracture, is not discussed in this book because it occurs much more often in contact sports and always requires a physician's care.

Once you're familiar with the common injury conditions, you'll be better prepared to move on to the specific injuries discussed in chapter 6. However, some basic information does not qualify you as a sports medicine expert. Use this information primarily as a means to *prevent* injury. If you do get hurt, use common sense when it comes to treating yourself and seeking treatment. You may not need a physician, but it always helps to seek the advice of your coaches and athletic trainers.

Abrasions

Definition: Abrasions also are known as "brush burns" or "raspberries." Abrasions result from the outer layers of skin being scraped off without penetration of the inner layers. A superficial wound results that is usually characterized by minimal bleeding and substantial amounts of imbedded dirt.

Cause: Baseball players suffer abrasions when they slide into a base or fall while fielding a ball. The skin rubs over the rough ground, and abrasions result.

Treatment: Immediate first aid for an abrasion requires the injury to be thoroughly rinsed with water to remove all foreign debris. After rinsing, wash the injured area with soap and water. Finally, rinse the wound again, but this time use hydrogen peroxide instead of water. To prevent infection, apply an antibiotic ointment evenly over the abrasion and then lightly cover the wound with gauze. The gauze cover will also keep your clothes from rubbing the wound and causing unnecessary irritation. Be sure to remove the gauze every evening so that the injury can dry completely.

Blisters

Definition: Blisters are abnormal pockets of tissue fluids between the outer and inner surfaces of the skin. The outer skin layer is the blister's covering. The inner layers of blistered skin are red and raw. Although most blisters are small and minor injuries, they can be quite bothersome and painful and often impede the capabilities of an affected player.

Cause: Blisters often are associated with preseason activities. An athlete's skin is not yet toughened by the rigors of the game and becomes raw from repeated rubbing between the skin and baseball gloves, balls, bats, and cleats.

Treatment: Treatment begins by cleansing the affected area with rubbing alcohol. Next, puncture the blister's edge with a sterilized needle. Drain the blister fluid by applying pressure to the wound with a sterile gauze pad. Then apply an antibiotic ointment evenly over the blister and cover the area with a pressure pad to prevent the blister from refilling with fluid. If the outer layer of skin has been torn, the wound should be treated as an abrasion. Cleanse the wound thoroughly with soap and water and then rinse it with hydrogen peroxide. If the outer layer of skin is still intact, lay it back over the injury. Without that outer layer, the wound will be far more susceptible to infection. Next apply an even layer of antibiotic ointment over the blister, and cover the area with a sterile dressing. After several days, you can remove the dead skin with scissors. Do not tear it off.

Prevention: Blisters can be easily prevented by wearing extra padding in body areas most likely to form blisters. Wear a batter's glove during batting practice. Apply strips of elastic tape over friction points of your throwing hand. Wear two pairs of socks while you're breaking in your cleats. "Wool over cotton" socks or tubular double knit socks are recommended.

Contusions

Definition: Contusions are more commonly known as "bruises" to the skin, muscles, and bones. When body tissues are crushed, blood vessels are ruptured, and blood flows into the surrounding tissues. This results in the "black and blue" marks so characteristic of contusions. The amount of bleeding depends upon the severity of the injury. Swelling may be evident immediately or as long as 24–48 hours after the injury has occurred.

Cause: Severe blows to the body are the most common cause of contusions. The force of the impact crushes tissues and blood vessels, and a contusion results. Although contusions are sustained most often in contact sports, baseball players also suffer contusions when they collide with each other during the game. Batters may suffer contusions when they are hit by a pitched ball.

Treatment: Contusions must be treated immediately. If ignored, swelling will soon limit the injured muscle's range of motion. First, stretch the affected muscle to its fullest range of motion. Then apply cold to the injured area in the form of an ice bag or a cold pack. Next apply a pressure dressing through the use of an elastic ace wrap bandage. This "stretch, cold, and compression" treatment must be repeated three to four times a day for the first 48 hours after the injury has occurred. If tenderness, pain, and restricted muscle movement persist, then continue the treatment for as long as necessary. Avoid using any form of heat (massages, whirlpools, or heating pads) on a contusion. Heat encourages the ruptured blood vessels to bleed even more profusely, thereby increasing the swelling. This prevents healing and can even lead to a far more serious condition. Icing a contused muscle in the stretched position is essential. Without the stretching, the affected muscle will contract and then tighten. Once the muscle has healed, you'll be left with an atrophied muscle that will require weeks of rehabilitation to return to good shape. Why wait longer than necessary to play baseball? Stretch initially and start playing sooner!

A *quadriceps contusion* or "charley horse" is the most prevalent form of contusion injury. Treatment must be immediate and requires you to stretch the affected front thigh muscle by bending your knee as far as possible. The easiest way to bend your knee is to sit on your heels. Next place a bag of ice over the stretched thigh for 15 minutes. Finally, secure an ace wrap bandage around the thigh to prevent further swelling.

Lacerations

Definition: A laceration is a deep cut that penetrates the outer and inner layers of the skin and sometimes the underlying tissues such as muscles, tendons, nerves, and blood vessels. The intensity of the bleeding depends on the severity of the wound.

Cause: Lacerations are generally caused by a player's impact with a sharp object. Basemen are especially vulnerable as they risk collision with sharp baseball cleats whenever a runner slides into their bases.

Treatment: Bleeding from a laceration must be stopped immediately. Next, cleanse the injured area thoroughly, taking care to prevent additional debris from entering the wound. Apply a dry, sterile dressing to reduce the risk of further contamination. Many lacerations require the care of a physician, who may have to suture the injury to ensure permanent healing.

Ligament Sprains

Definition: Ligament sprains are an overstretching, partial tear, or complete rupture of the fibrous tissues or *ligaments* that connect bones to bones and that support and strengthen joints. One of the most common sports injuries, sprains are divided into three classifications, including mild (first degree sprain), moderate (second degree sprain), and severe (third degree sprain).

Cause: Sprains occur when ligaments are stretched beyond their strength capabilities. In baseball, sprains can occur during sudden changes of direction on the base path, by slipping on or catching your foot on a base, through strong impact between a limb and a hard object, or by abrupt and stressful twisting or turning motions.

Treatment: Regardless of the severity of your injury, stop playing if you experience pain. Treat the injured area using the RICE principle (see chapter 4). If swelling or disability occurs, visit a sports medicine physician as soon as possible. The rehabilitative exercises you'll find in chapter 6 are a major part of the treatment of ligament sprains. Although the injured ligament may require 6–8 weeks to heal, the rehabilitative exercises will increase the strength and flexibility of muscles and tendons surrounding the ligament. These muscles and tendons will then substitute for the injured ligament in its role of supporting and strengthening the joints and bones it connects. As a result, players do not have to wait 6–8 weeks to return to competition. Instead, they return much sooner, fully capable of playing their best game. Statistics indicate that baseball players suffer most of their sprains in the ankles, knees, and fingers. Young players must be especially careful to avoid sprains. Children's growing bones are often weaker than the ligaments that support them. When a ligament is overstretched, it may yank so hard on a bone growth site that the bone will break before the ligament tears.

Muscle Strains

Definition: When a muscle is stretched beyond its range of motion capability, a strain results. The muscle is pulled or torn, and the injured athlete suffers persistent pain in the muscle that has been over-exerted. Many athletes make the mistake of continuing to compete despite the strain. All they achieve is reduced playing capability, further muscle damage, and a prolonged healing period.

Cause: Muscle strains have numerous causes. Many players, for example, do not warm up their muscles sufficiently before exercising or playing. They play with cold, stiff muscles that are not as flexible as they would be if athletes took the time to warm them up. Other players seldom, if ever, stretch. Their muscles are so contracted and inflexible that they are bound to be strained during competition. Poor training can lead to strains. Training itself must be challenging enough to prepare you for the rigors of your game. Another cause of muscle strain is imbalance between partner muscles. Whenever one of your muscles contracts, its partner muscle—or antagonist—relaxes. Partner muscles should be equally strong. When one is stronger, it places unnecessary stress on the other. As a result, the weaker muscle tears.

Treatment: Muscle strains should be treated immediately using the RICE principle (see chapter 4). Continue RICE for at least 48–72 hours. Begin rehabilitative exercises at the end of the first week. The exercises should be specific to the muscle injured and should aid the restoration of balance between muscle strength and muscle flexibility.

Tendonitis

Definition: Tendonitis is an inflammation of the tissues or *tendons* that connect muscles to bones and cartilage. Athletes with tendonitis suffer swelling and pain in the affected area.

Cause: Tendonitis results from the prolonged misuse of the connecting tissues. When muscles are contracted suddenly, they tug the tendons. This tugging force is increased whenever unstretched, improperly trained muscles are too inflexible to extend to the full range of motion needed for competition. In the process of "overstretching" tight muscles, you create tiny tears in the tendons. Continued abuse of torn tendons results in tendonitis. Pitchers, who must throw repetitively, are especially susceptible to this ailment.

Treatment: Treatment of tendonitis begins with the application of an ice bag or an ice massage to the injured area. In addition, the players *must rest* the injured tendon for at least several days. Once the pain has subsided, begin a regular program of rehabilitative stretching exercises.

Chapter
6

Baseball's Most
Commonly
Used and
Injured Muscles

You cannot fully appreciate your muscles when you know little or nothing about them. You take care of what you value; what you know nothing about or consider unimportant, you neglect.

Don't neglect your muscles! Muscle health is essential to your success in baseball. You don't have to become an exercise physiology expert or sports medicine specialist, but you do need some basic knowledge about what muscles you are working, where they're located, and how they connect to the rest of your body.

Take the time to review the illustrations in this chapter. The muscles depicted are the ones you as a baseball player will use most often and are thus most likely to injure. If you play a position that demands a great deal from certain muscles, then take special care of those muscles. And as you play, visualize your muscles in action as they stretch and then contract.

What you understand you will be able to appreciate. Appreciating your muscles will result in less pain, less injury, and more hours participating in the sport that has attracted countless fans over the years.

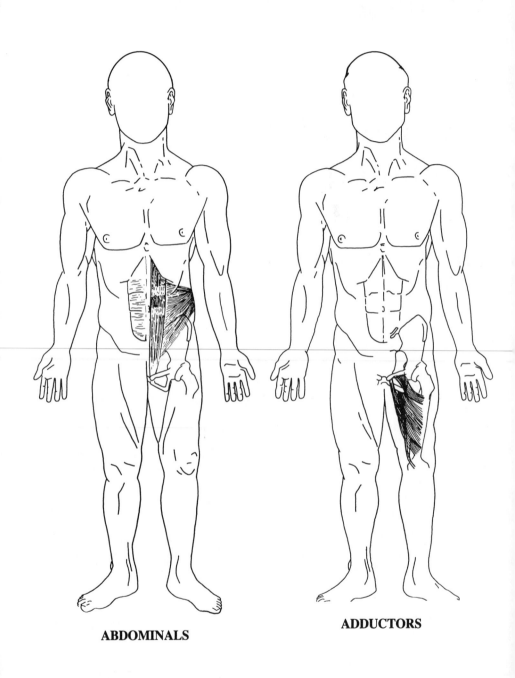

ABDOMINALS

ADDUCTORS

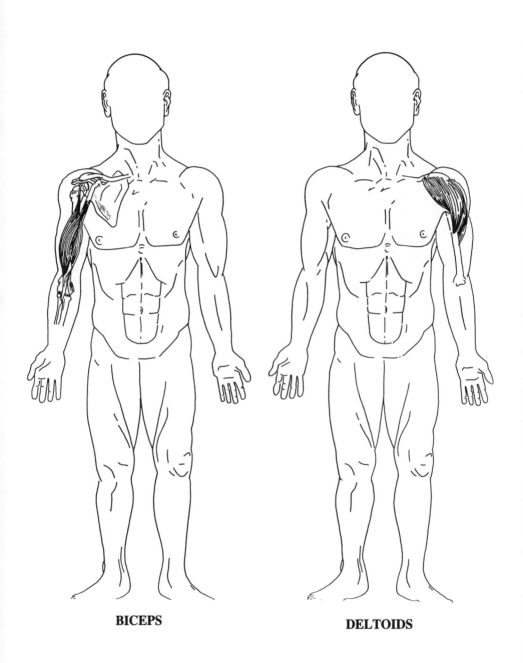

BICEPS   **DELTOIDS**

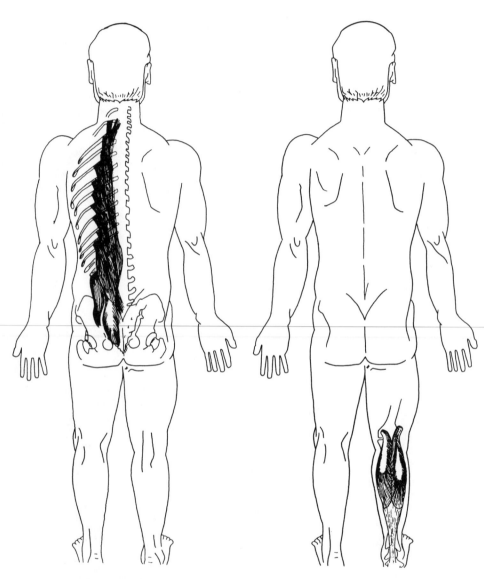

ERECTOR SPINAE   **GASTROCNEMIUS**

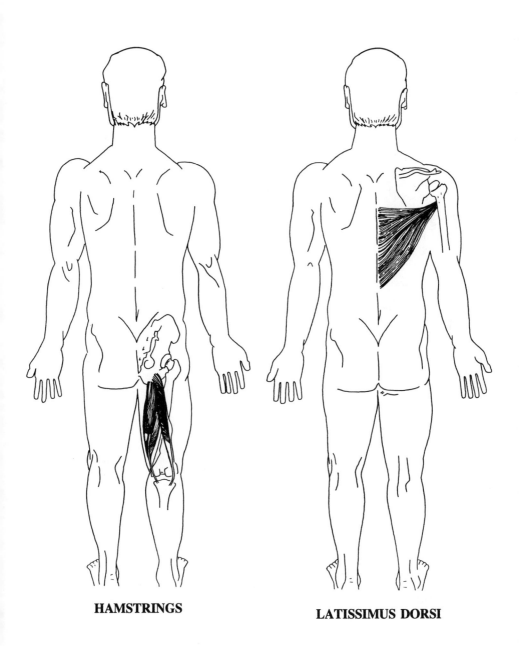

HAMSTRINGS   **LATISSIMUS DORSI**

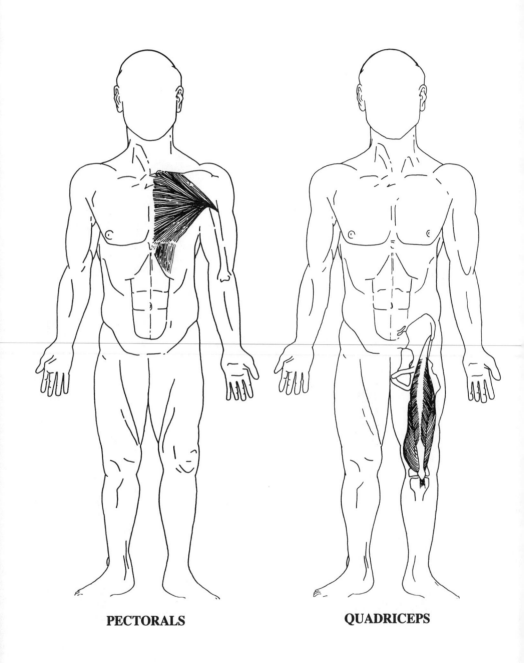

PECTORALS   **QUADRICEPS**

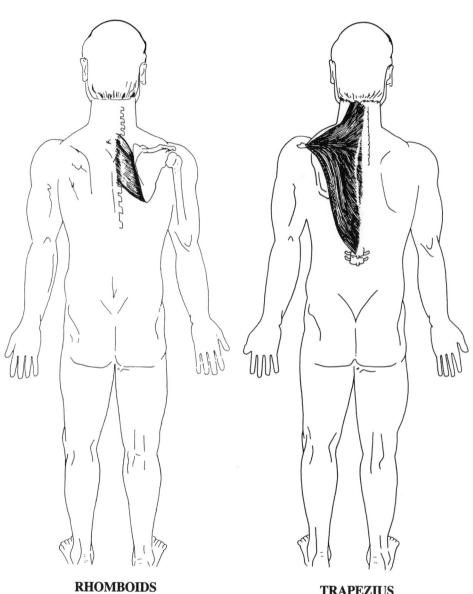

RHOMBOIDS   **TRAPEZIUS**

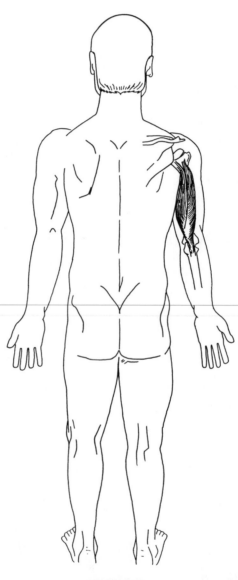

TRICEPS

Chapter 7

Treatment of Baseball Injuries

Today, as in the past, baseball injuries are bound to occur. The sport is aggressive, and each game is intense. A good player will often risk bodily health to snag a fly ball or steal just one more base.

But today's players, unlike their counterparts of earlier years, recover from injuries more rapidly with less chance for injuries to recur. Why the improvement? Because aggressiveness on the field is treated off the field with equally aggressive sports medicine philosophy.

It's about time.

Gone are the days when injuries meant long periods of immobilization and inactivity. Although athletes may have to refrain from playing baseball until their injuries have healed, they don't have to give up exercising. Instead, sports medicine specialists encourage injured players to continue working out during periods of rehabilitation. By maintaining their overall fitness and flexibility, players return to competition in excellent shape instead of out-of-shape from weeks of inactivity.

Out-of-shape players get reinjured. Conditioned players give top performances—and win games.

In addition to insisting upon ongoing conditioning programs, sports medicine specialists give players specific instructions for strengthening, stretching, supporting, and protecting injured muscles and joints. Only in extreme cases is immobilization prescribed. Although injured limbs will heal if kept motionless, they will heal in an atrophied, weakened condition and will require more extensive rehabilitation before active play can resume.

Why wait? Injured muscles can be stretched and strengthened *as* they heal instead of *after* they heal. Injured areas can be taped and protected so that exercise programs can continue without aggravating injuries.

Treatment begins with a sound philosophy. Sports medicine is it.

The sports medicine treatments presented in this chapter are ones that I use regularly for both professional and amateur athletes. Each injury discussed includes information on causes and symptoms. Depending on the condition, you'll find instructions for taping techniques, selecting the best possible protective supports, and stretching and strengthening the injured muscles and ligaments.

All the injuries described are on the right side of the body. Should you injure your left side, just reverse the instructions where necessary.

For best results, perform your rehabilitation exercises twice daily. Each stretch should be held for 10 seconds and repeated five times. The strengthening exercises require very specific repetitions and holding times.

As you perform the exercises, don't get lazy. It's easy to convince yourself that a sequence of four stretches is as effective as a sequence of five, that 20 strengthening repetitions will do the job as well as 30 repetitions. The more you avoid helping your body get better, the more time your body will need to heal itself. It's that simple. So don't be lazy.

In learning the taping techniques, remember that practice makes perfect. If you tape properly, you ensure maximum support for your injured limb. Carefully follow the step-by-step instructions and accompanying illustrations. Tape yourself for practice whenever possible or tape another player or a friend. As you practice, be careful to smooth out all the wrinkles in the tape itself. Bunched tape will rub against the skin and cause blisters. Tape properly and you will avoid causing a second injury while trying to rehabilitate the first one.

Those of you who have some familiarity with sports medicine will notice I neglect to recommend the use of aspirin for injuries that are inflamed or swollen. Aspirin is an inexpensive, easily obtainable, and highly effective pain killer and anti-inflammatory agent. I advise my patients who are not allergic to aspirin to take eight aspirins a day (two every four hours) until the swelling and pain disappear. Many sports medicine specialists believe that taking aspirin is as vital a part of the treatment as the rehabilitative exercises.

Why, then, have I failed to mention aspirin when I describe different treatments? Because aspirin is a *medication*. Because it's easy to obtain, it's easy to abuse. In addition, some athletes are allergic to aspirin or should not take it for other medical reasons. The best advice I can give you is to take aspirin when you need it but to take it with care. If the injury is swollen or inflamed enough to require aspirin, it should be examined by a qualified physician who can work with you to develop a rehabilitation program best suited to your injury needs.

Remember that your coaches and your trainers are often your best sources of advice about the injuries you may receive as you compete. If you get hurt, tell them. Don't try to hide an injury and rehabilitate yourself on the sly while you continue to play. Baseball is a team game. Be a good team player by confessing your injury so that you can receive the treatment you need to recover fully and resume your role.

Achilles Tendonitis

Symptoms: Tenderness in the region of the Achilles tendon located between the calf muscle (gastrocnemius) and heel bone (calcaneus); pain experienced with ankle motion.

Causes: Overuse or overstretching of the Achilles tendon; commonly results from sport activities requiring quick bursts of speed such as sprinting from the batter's box.

Protective Support: Insert a quarter-inch felt or rubber heel lift into the heels of both your cleats and your street shoes. The heel lift will elevate your heel, thereby reducing the stress on the Achilles tendon.

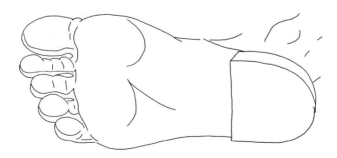

Achilles Tendonitis

Rehabilitative Exercise #1

Stand erect and face a wall or fence. Straighten your legs and place your heels flat on the ground. Slowly lean forward at the hips. If necessary, use your arms for support.

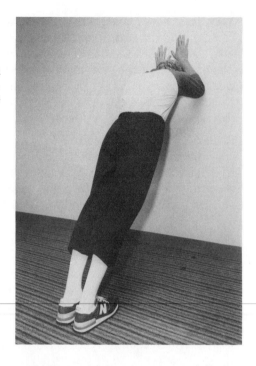

Achilles Tendonitis

Rehabilitative Exercise #2

Stand erect and face a wall or fence. Straighten your legs and place your heels flat on the ground. Slowly lean forward at the knees. If necessary, use your arms for support and be sure that your heels remain flat on the ground.

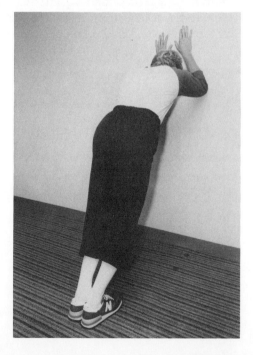

Bicipital Tendonitis

Symptoms: Tenderness in the region of the biceps tendon located in the front of the shoulder; pain experienced with shoulder motion.

Causes: Overuse or misuse of the shoulder. Bicipital tendonitis is a thrower's ailment and is especially prevalent among repetitive throwers such as baseball pitchers.

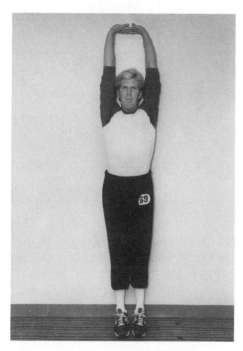

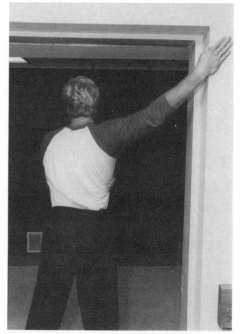

Bicipital Tendonitis

Rehabilitative Exercise #1

Stand erect. Raise your arms above your head and interlock your fingers. Straighten your arms and then turn your palms forward and upward. Slowly pull your arms backward.

Bicipital Tendonitis

Rehabilitative Exercise #2

Stand erect and rest your right hand on a doorjamb. Straighten your right arm and then grasp the right side of your rib cage with your left hand. Slowly lean forward through the doorway. At the same time, pull your trunk to the left.

Bicipital Tendonitis

Rehabilitative Exercise #3

Stand erect and place the back of your right arm flat against a doorjamb. Bend your left arm behind your head and grasp your right wrist with your left hand. Slowly lean forward through the doorway. At the same time, push your right hand away from your head.

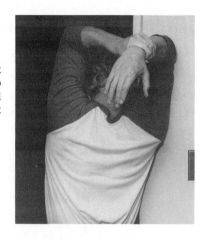

Bunions

Symptoms: Tenderness at the base of the great toe; pain experienced during walking or running.

Causes: The result of cleats that are too narrow or too short, thereby causing the great toe to angle inward toward the other toes.

Protective Support: Wear properly fitted shoes and cleats that do not cramp the toes. In addition, create a wedge between the great toe and the second toe by inserting a quarter-inch piece of felt.

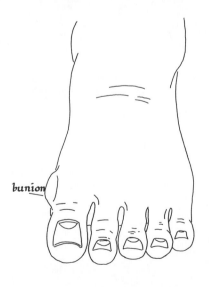

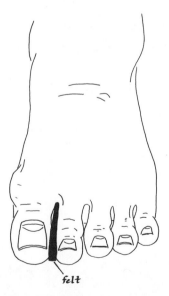

Charley Horse (Quadriceps Contusion)

Symptoms: Tenderness in the region of the front thigh (quadriceps); pain experienced with knee motion.

Causes: Trauma or blows to the thigh, such as being hit by a baseball. The blow results in a contusion (bruise) to the muscle.

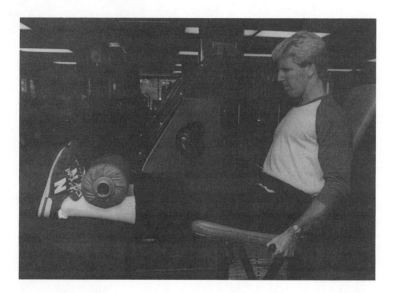

Charley Horse

Rehabilitative Exercise #1

For this exercise, use the Nautilus Leg Extension machine or some other form of resistance. Sit down and slowly extend your right leg until it is straight. Hold this position for 1 second and then repeat the exercise for 2 sets of 15 reps. Increase the weight as you build up your tolerance.

Charley Horse

Rehabilitative Exercise #2
Kneel so that the tops of your feet are flat on the ground. Slowly sit back on your heels.

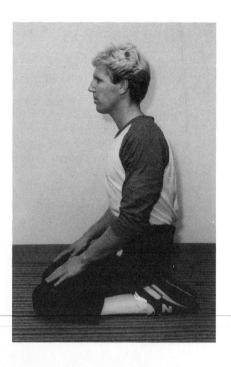

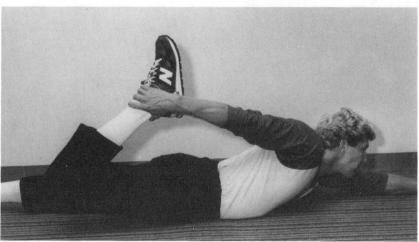

Charley Horse

Rehabilitative Exercise #3
Lie on your stomach. Bend your right knee and try to touch your right heel to your right buttock. Next grasp your right ankle with your right hand. Slowly pull your ankle toward the back of your head. Avoid twisting your trunk.

Groin Pull (Adductor Strain)

Symptoms: Tenderness in the region of the inside thigh (adductor).

Causes: Overstretching of the groin muscles resulting from activities such as sprinting around the base path.

Protective Support: Support the area by fitting the player with a PRO "Groin Strap"[1] or with a 4-inch elastic ace wrap bandage (hip spica procedure).

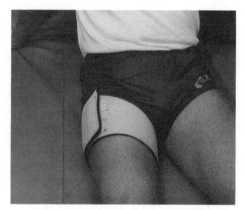

Groin Pull

Hip Spica Procedure
Materials: One roll of 4-inch elastic ace wrap bandage; one strip of 1-1/2-inch adhesive tape.

Position of Player: Stand erect and turn your injured leg slightly inward.

Procedure: As shown in Step #1, place the end of the 4-inch ace wrap bandage on the outside of your upper thigh. Wrap the bandage across the front of your upper thigh, between your legs, and around the back of your thigh. Then return to your starting point.

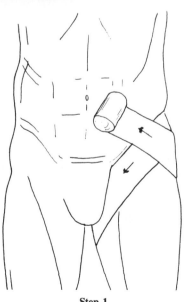

Step 1

[1]PRO Orthopedic Devices, Inc., P.O. Box 27525, Tucson, AZ 85726, (800) 523-5611

As shown in Step #2, next wrap the bandage across your lower abdomen, and around the hip of your uninjured leg, and around your lower back. Then return to your starting point.

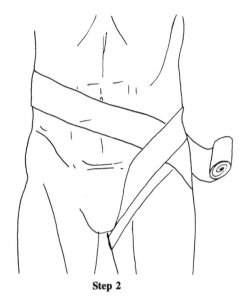

Step 2

As shown in Step #3, repeat the wrapping sequence outlined in Step #2 until you have used all the ace wrap bandage. Secure the bandage with a strip of 1-1/2-inch adhesive tape.

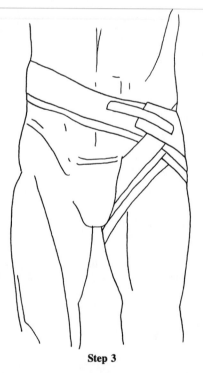

Step 3

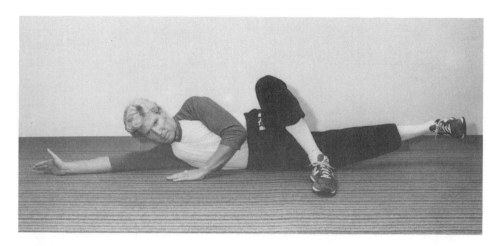

Groin Pull

Rehabilitative Exercise #1

Lie on your right side. Bend your left leg over your right leg and rest your left foot flat on the floor in front of your right knee. Keep your right leg straight and your right foot parallel to the floor. Slowly lift your right leg. Hold this position for 1 second and the repeat the exercise for 2 sets of 15 reps.

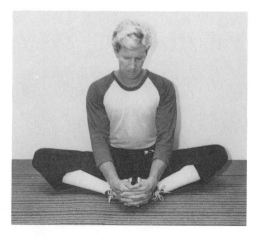

Groin Pull

Rehabilitative Exercise #2

Sit with your knees bent and with the soles of your feet together. Grasp your toes with both hands. Slowly pull your heels toward your groin. Use your hip muscles to slowly push your knees to the floor.

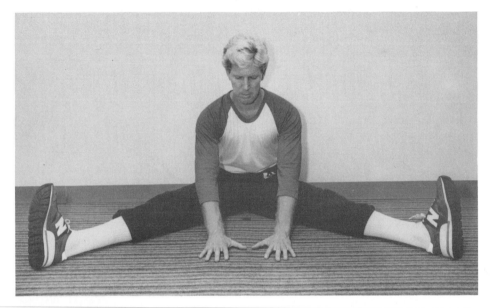

Groin Pull

Rehabilitative Exercise #3.
Sit with your legs spread wide apart. Slowly lean forward, keeping your legs straight.

Hamstring Pull (Hamstring Strain)

Symptoms: Tenderness in the region of the back thigh (hamstrings).

Causes: Weakness, inflexibility, fatigue, or overstretching of the hamstring. A common ailment of sprinters.

Protective Support: Support the affected area by fitting the player with a PRO "Thigh Sleeve."

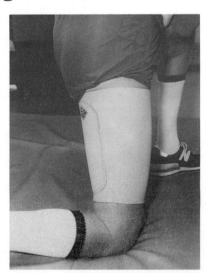

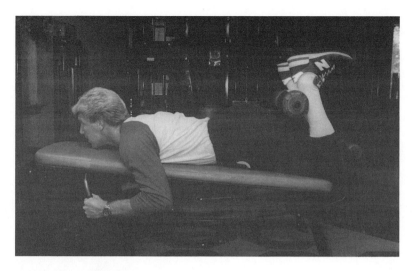

Hamstring Pull

Rehabilitative Exercise #1

For this exercise, use the Nautilus Leg Machine or some other form of resistance. Lie on your stomach and slowly curl your right heel toward your right buttock. Hold this position for 1 second and then repeat the exercise for 2 sets of 15 reps. Increase the weight as you build up your tolerance.

Hamstring Pull

Rehabilitative Exercise #2

Sit with your right leg straight. Bend your left leg so that your left foot slightly touches the inside of your right thigh. Slowly bend forward at the hips and try to touch your chin to your right foot.

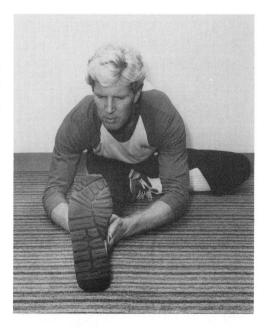

Hamstring Pull

Rehabilitative Exercise #3.
Sit with your legs straight. Slowly bend forward at
the hips and try to touch your chin to your toes.

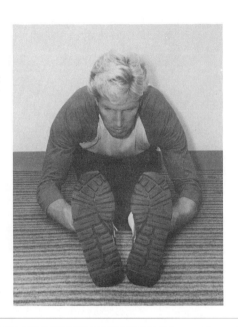

Heel Bruise (Calcaneal Contusion)

Symptoms: Tenderness over the bottom of the heel bone (calcaneus).

Causes: Contact between the heel and a hard surface resulting from traumas such
as running over a stone or touching a base heel first.

Protective Support: Protect the affected area with a heel cup or a quarter-inch felt
doughnut inserted into the heels of both cleats and street shoes.

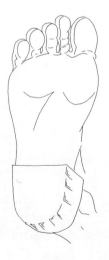

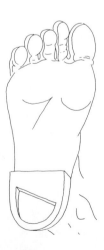

Ingrown Toenail

Symptoms: Irritation at the side and borders of a toenail.

Causes: Improper clipping of the toenail, poorly fitted cleats, getting stepped on by another player.

Protective Support: Wear properly fitted shoes and cleats that do not cramp the toes. In addition, cut a "V" shape into the center of the outer edge of your toenail.

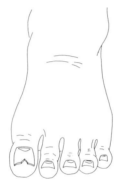

Leg Cramps

Symptoms: Pain in the calf (gastrocnemius) while at rest; usually occurs after activity.

Causes: Fatigue, inflexibility, weakness, or excess fluid loss due to perspiration.

Leg Cramps

Rehabilitative Exercise #1

Stand erect and face a wall or fence. Straighten your legs and place your heels flat on the ground. Slowly lean forward at the hips. If necessary, use your arms for support. Augment the benefits of this rehabilitative exercise by massaging your calf with an analgesic balm ointment.

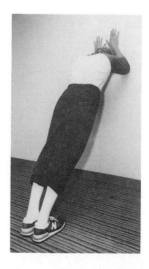

"Little League Elbow" (Medial Epicondyle Epiphysis Avulsion)

Symptoms: Tenderness at the knob of the inner elbow; most commonly affects young baseball players between 8–16 years of age.

Causes: "Little league elbow" is a thrower's ailment caused by the forceful stress placed on the elbow during a throw or pitch. In children, the elbow is the site of the growth center, which is weak and therefore even more affected by the force of a pitch.

Rehabilitative Exercises: The following exercises for "little league elbow" should be performed only after X-ray findings and your family physician's evaluation indicate that your elbow has healed.

Little League Elbow

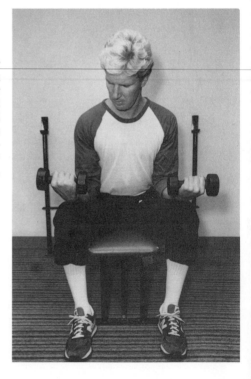

Rehabilitative Exercise #1

Sit in a chair. Bend your knees and place your feet flat on the floor. Place your right forearm on your right thigh. Your wrist should hang over your knee. Bend your elbow at a 90°angle and position your hand "palm up." Make a fist and slowly pull your right hand upward. Hold this position for 1 second and then repeat the exercise for 2 sets of 15 reps. Begin this exercise by using no weight. You may add weight, however, as you build up your tolerance.

Little League Elbow

Rehabilitative Exercise #2

Sit in a chair. Bend your knees and place your feet flat on the floor. Place your right forearm on your right thigh. Your wrist should hang over your knee. Bend your elbow at a 90°angle. Begin the exercise with your right hand in a "palm up" position. Using a dumbbell with the weight on one end of the bar only, slowly rotate your right hand counterclockwise until your hand is in a "palm down" position. Hold this position for 1 second and then repeat the exercise for 2 sets of 15 reps. Use a light weight initially and increase the weight as you build up your tolerance. This exercise also can be made more challenging by grasping the dumbbell farther away from the weights.

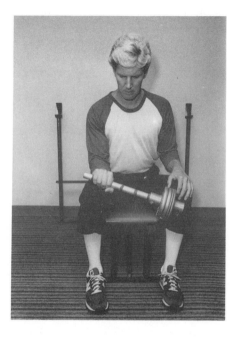

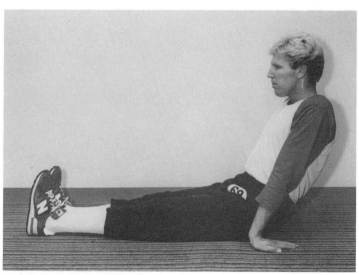

Little League Elbow

Rehabilitative Exercise #3

Sit on the floor. Place your palms flat on the floor by your sides. Point your thumbs outward and your fingers backward. Straighten your elbows and then slowly lean backward.

Low Back Strain

Symptoms: Tenderness and lack of mobility of the low back muscles (erector spinae).

Causes: Poor body mechanics, inflexibility, fatigue, or weakness.

Protective Support: Support the affected area with a Jerome "Low Back Support."[2]

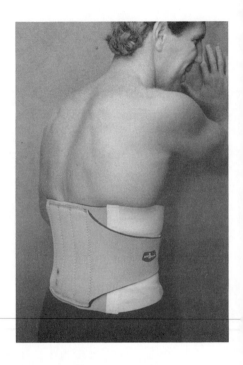

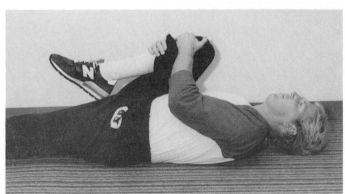

Low Back Strain

Rehabilitative Exercise #1

Lie flat on your back. Grasp your right knee with your hands and slowly pull your knee toward your chest. Hold this position for 10 seconds and then repeat the exercise five times. Next, grasp your left knee with your hands and perform the entire exercise again.

[2]Jerome Medical, 309 Fellowship Road, Mt. Laurel, NJ 08054, (800) 257-8440

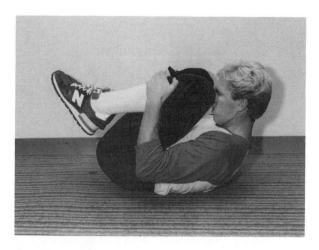

Low Back Strain

Rehabilitative Exercise #2

Lie flat on your back. Bend your knees and place your feet flat on the floor. Grab your knees with your hands and slowly pull your knees toward your chest. At the same time curl your head toward your knees.

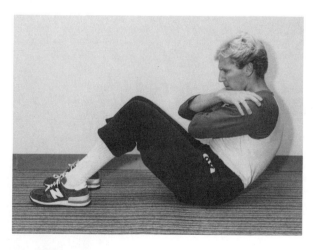

Low Back Strain

Rehabilitative Exercise #3

Lie flat on your back. Bend your knees and place your feet on the floor. Grab your shoulders with the opposite hands. Slowly tighten your abdominal muscles and then sit up as far as possible. Hold this position for 1 second and then repeat the exercise as many times as you can. Gradually increase your strength until you can repeat the exercise 30 times without stopping.

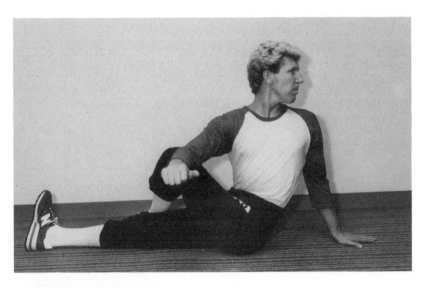

Low Back Strain

Rehabilitative Exercise #4

Sit with your right leg straight. Bend your left leg over your right leg and place your left foot flat on the floor on the outside of your right knee. Touch your right elbow to the outside of your left knee. Place your left hand on the floor behind you. Slowly look over your left shoulder and rotate your trunk to the left. At the same time, apply counterpressure to your left knee with your right elbow. Hold this position for 10 seconds, then repeat the exercise five times. Reverse leg positions and stretch to the other side.

Low Back Strain

Rehabilitative Exercise #5

Sit in a chair. Spread your legs apart with your feet flat on the floor. Grab your elbows with the opposite hands. Slowly lean forward between your legs as far as you can. Hold this position for 1 second, then return to a sitting position for 1 second. Repeat the exercise for 2 sets of 15 reps.

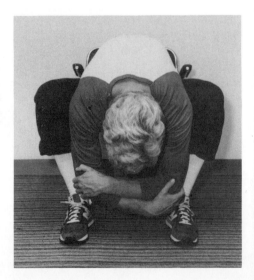

"Pitcher's Elbow"

Symptoms: Tenderness at the knob of the inner elbow; pain experienced in straightening the elbows.

Causes: Stress placed on the elbow from the force generated by a throw or a pitch. Repetitive throwers such as pitchers are especially vulnerable.

Protective Support: Support the affected areas with a PRO "Elbow Sleeve" or a Jerome "Pitcher's Strap."

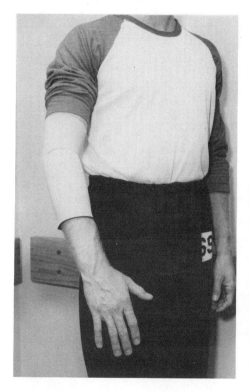
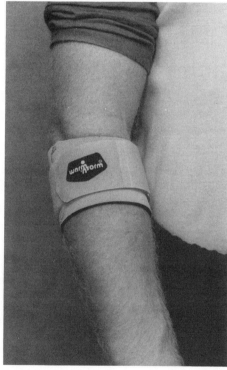

Pitcher's Elbow

Rehabilitative Exercise #1

Stand erect. Raise your arms above your head and interlock your fingers. Straighten your arms and then turn your palms forward and upward. Slowly pull your arms backward.

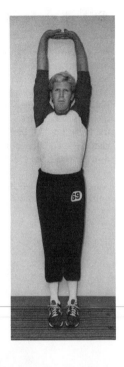

Pitcher's Elbow

Rehabilitative Exercise #2

Sit in a chair. Bend your knees and place your feet flat on the floor. Place your right forearm on your right thigh. Your wrist should hang over your knee. Bend your elbow at a 90°angle and position your hand "palm up." Make a fist and slowly pull your right hand upward. Hold this position for 1 second and then repeat the exercise for 2 sets of 15 reps. Begin this exercise by using no weight. You may add weight, however, as you build up your tolerance.

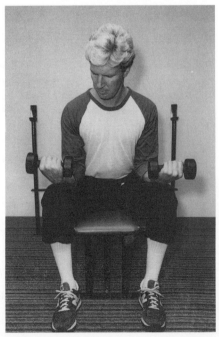

Pitcher's Elbow

Rehabilitative Exercise #3

Sit in a chair. Bend your knees and place your feet flat on the floor. Place your right forearm on your right thigh. Your wrist should hang over your knee. Bend your elbow at a 90° angle. Begin the exercise with your right hand in a "palm up" position. Using a dumbbell with the weight on one end of the bar only, slowly rotate your right hand counterclockwise until your hand is in a "palm down" position. Hold this position for 1 second, then repeat the exercise for 2 sets of 15 reps. Use a light weight initially and increase the weight as you build up your tolerance. This exercise can also be made more challenging by grasping the dumbbell farther away from the weights.

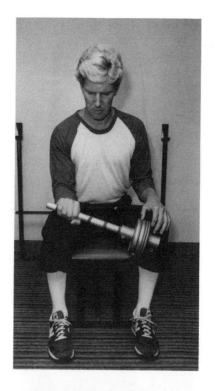

Pitcher's Elbow

Rehabilitative Exercise #4

Grasp a rubber ball or a PRO "Sports Grip" with your right hand. Squeeze the ball or grip and concentrate on contracting your forearm muscles. Hold the contraction for 1 second and then repeat the exercise 30 times.

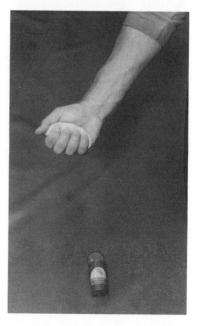

"Pitcher's Shoulder" (Rotator Cuff Strain)

Symptoms: Tenderness and lack of mobility of the shoulder.

Causes: Overuse or overstretching of the shoulder's rotary muscles used in the throwing motion; improper warm-up, inflexibility, and fatigue.

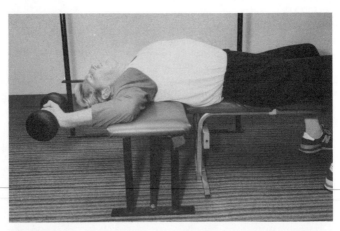

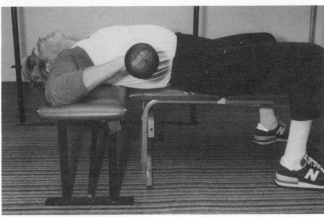

Pitcher's Shoulder

Rehabilitative Exercise #1

Lie flat on your back. Place your right elbow on the floor at shoulder level and bend it at a 90° angle. Grasp a light-weight dumbbell with your right hand. Slowly pull your forearm backward until the back of your right hand touches the floor. Hold this position for 1 second. Reverse direction until the palm of your right hand touches the floor. Hold this position for 1 second, then repeat the entire exercise for 2 sets of 15 reps. Increase the weight as you build up your tolerance.

Pitcher's Shoulder

Rehabilitative Exercise #2

Stand erect. Bend your right arm at a 90°angle and place the arm in front of you. Face your right palm toward your body. Bend your left arm underneath your right arm and grasp your right thumb with your left hand. Slowly pull your right arm down to the floor.

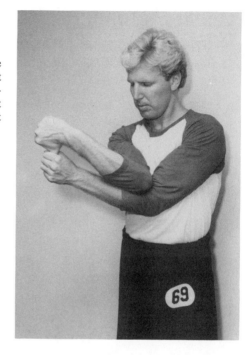

Pitcher's Shoulder

Rehabilitative Exercise #3

Stand erect and bend your right arm behind your head. Grasp your right elbow with your left hand and slowly pull your elbow away from your head.

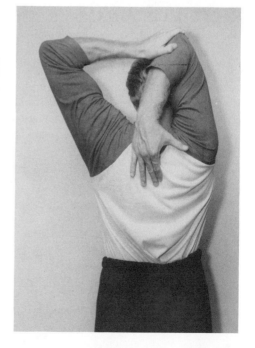

Pitcher's Shoulder

Rehabilitative Exercise #4

Stand erect, and place the inside of your right upper arm against a doorjamb. Bend your elbow at a 90°angle and place it at shoulder level. Slowly lean forward through the doorjamb.

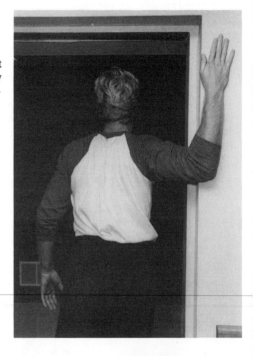

Sprained Ankle

Symptoms: Tenderness and swelling of the outer (lateral) portion of the ankle.

Causes: Sudden, abnormal twisting or turning of the ankle until the ankle bone is forced away from the ankle joint; caused by traumas such as slipping or tripping on a base.

Protective Support: Support the affected area with a PRO "Ankle Support" or with "basketweave" ankle taping.

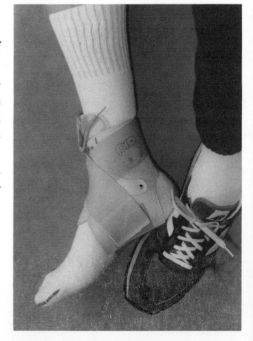

Sprained Ankle

"Basketweave" Ankle Taping

Materials: One roll of 1-1/2-inch adhesive tape; two lubricated 4 by 4-inch gauze pads.

Position of Player: Sit down, place your injured foot in front of you, and bend your ankle up toward your body.

Procedure: As shown in Step #1, place one lubricated 4 x 4-inch gauze pad over your instep. Place the other pad above your heel bone. Wrap one anchor strip of 1-1/2-inch adhesive tape around your leg below the base of the calf (a). Wrap a second anchor strip around the arch of your foot and then around your leg just above your ankle bone (b).

As shown in Step #2, attach a stirrup strip to the top anchor over the inside of your leg. Place the strip down the length of your ankle behind the ankle bone. Wrap it under your heel and up the outside of your leg. Attach the stirrup strip to the top anchor (c). Attach a horseshoe strip to the inside of the arch anchor. Wrap the strip below the ankle bone, around the heel, and to the other side of your foot. Attach the strip to the outside of the arch anchor (d).

As shown in Step #3, alternate two additional stirrup tapings (e and g) with two additional horseshoe tapings (f and h). Overlap each of the strips in the second layer over just half of their related strips in the first layer.

As shown in Step #4, continue applying horseshoe strips up your ankle until you reach the top anchor. Make two final anchor strips. Wrap one strip around your leg below the base of the calf (i). Wrap the second strip around the arch of your foot and then around your leg just above your ankle bone (j).

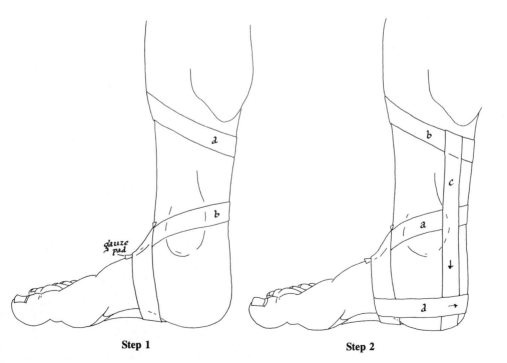

Step 1   Step 2

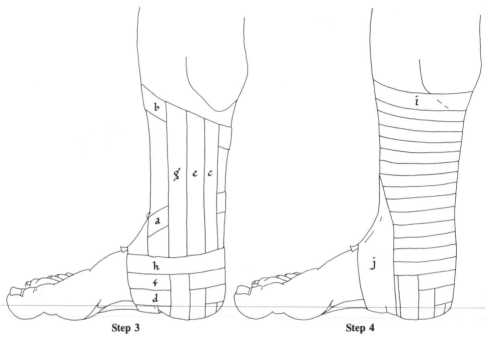

Step 3   Step 4

Sprained Ankle

Rehabilitative Exercise #1

Stand erect and face a wall. Straighten your legs and place your heels flat on the floor. Slowly lean forward at the hip. If necessary, use your arms for support.

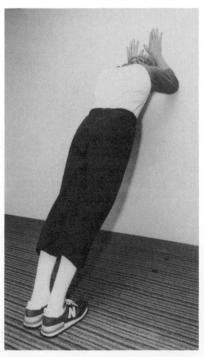

Sprained Ankle

Rehabilitative Exercise #2

Stand erect and face a wall. Straighten your legs and place
your heels flat on the floor. Slowly bend forward at the knees.
If necessary, use your arms for support.

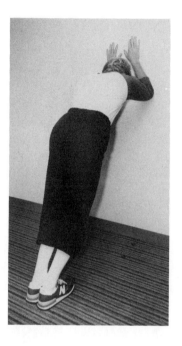

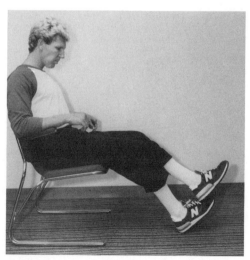

Sprained Ankle

Rehabilitative Exercise #3

Sit with your left heel on top of your right foot. Slowly pull your right foot upward. At the same
time, apply resistance by pushing downward with your left heel. Maintain the resistance for 1 second, then repeat the exercise for 2 sets of 15 reps.

Sprained Ankle

Rehabilitative Exercise #4
Sit with your left foot crossed behind your right foot. Slowly rotate your right foot to the right. At the same time, apply resistance by rotating your left foot to the left. Maintain the resistance for 1 second and then repeat the exercise for 2 sets of 15 reps.

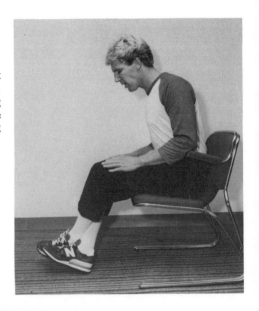

Sprained Finger (Jammed Finger)

Symptoms: Tenderness and swelling of a finger joint.

Causes: Strong impact at the fingertip caused by catching a baseball barehanded, sliding into a base hands-first, etc.

Protective Support: Support the affected area with "buddy" finger taping.

Sprained Finger

"Buddy" Finger Taping
Materials: One roll of half-inch adhesive tape; one 4 x 4-inch gauze pad.

Position of Player: Hold your injured index finger in a relaxed fashion.

Procedure: As shown in Step #1, using a 4 x 4-inch gauze pad, cut a gauze strip the size of your index finger's width. Place the strip between your index and middle fingers in order to prevent rubbing and the formation of blisters.

As shown in Step #2, wrap a strip of half-inch adhesive tape around the bases of the index and middle fingers (a). Then wrap a second strip of tape just above the fingers' middle knuckles (b).

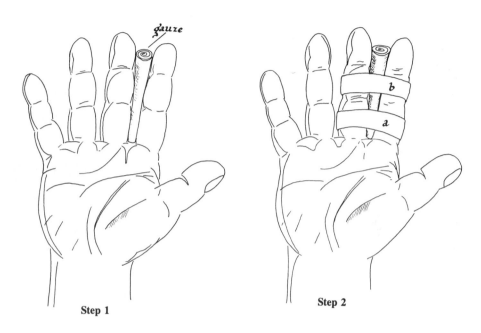

Step 1

Step 2

Sprained Great Toe

Symptoms: Tenderness at the base of the great toe.

Causes: Swift changes in direction caused by rounding the bases on an extra-base hit, etc.

Protective Support: Support the affected area with "turf toe" taping.

Sprained Great Toe

"Turf Toe" Taping

Materials: One roll of 1-inch adhesive tape, one 4 x 4-inch gauze pad.

Position of Player: Sit down, place your injured foot in front of you, and relax your great toe.

Procedure: As shown in Step #1, using a 4 x 4-inch gauze pad, cut a gauze strip the size of your great toe's width. Place the strip between your great toe and your second toe in order to prevent rubbing and the formation of blisters. Wrap an anchor strip of 1-inch adhesive tape around the arch of your foot (a).

As shown in Step #2, attach a stirrup strip to the top of the anchor strip. Place the stirrup strip along the top length of your great toe, wrap it around the front of your toe, and place it along the toe's lower length. Attach the end of the stirrup strip to the bottom of the anchor strip (b). For additional support, place a second stirrup strip on top of the first stirrup strip. Wrap the second stirrup strip around your great toe in the same way (c). Next wrap another strip of tape around the bases of the great and second toes (d). To secure all the strips, wrap a final anchor strip around the arch of your foot (e). As it's being taped, your great toe should be kept straight and relaxed.

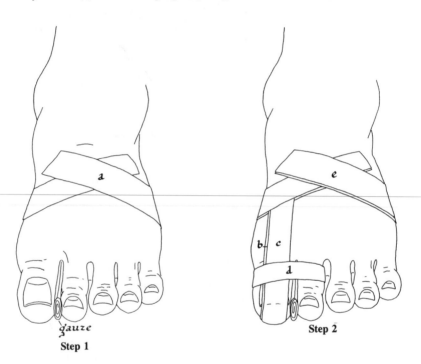

gauze

Step 1

Step 2

Sprained Knee

Symptoms: Tenderness or swelling of the inside (medial) or of the outside (lateral) areas of the knee.

Causes: Sudden twisting or overextension of the knee caused by twisting the leg to the side to field a ground ball or similar traumas.

Protective Support: Support the affected area with a PRO "Knee Brace" or with "collateral" knee taping.

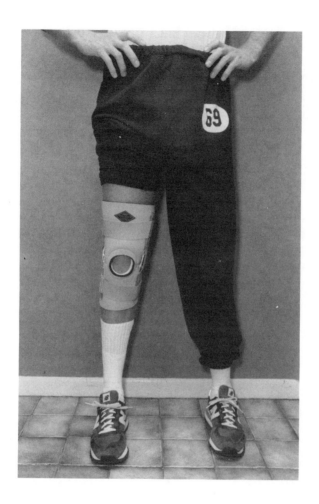

Sprained Knee

"Collateral" Knee Taping

Materials: One roll of 2-inch adhesive tape; one roll of 3-inch elastic stretch tape.

Position of Player: Stand erect and rest the heel of your injured leg on a 2-inch high board or roll of tape or other support. This position places the affected knee in a relaxed degree of flexion.

Procedure: As shown in Step #1, wrap an anchor strip of 2-inch adhesive tape around the middle of the thigh (a). Wrap a second anchor strip around the base of your calf (b). Next use 3-inch elastic stretch tape to make collateral strips. Attach the first strip to the calf anchor along the inside of your calf. Wrap the strip across the lower leg and upward to the outside of the upper leg. Attach the strip to the thigh anchor (c). Attach the second collateral strip to the calf anchor along the outside of your calf. Wrap this strip across the lower leg and upward to the inside of your upper leg. Attach the strip to the thigh anchor (d). Attach the third collateral strip to the first collateral strip along the inside of your calf. Place the strip up the inner length of your lower leg, and then cross the strip above your kneecap to the outside of your upper leg. Attach the strip to the thigh anchor (e). Attach the fourth collateral strip to the second collateral strip along the outside of your calf. Place the strip up the outer length of your lower leg and then cross the strip above your kneecap to the inside of your upper leg. Attach the strip to the thigh anchor (f).

As shown in Step #2, repeat each collateral taping (g, h, i, j), overlapping each of the strips in the second layer over just half of their related strips in the first layer.

As shown in Step #3, use a 3-inch elastic stretch tape to make two final anchor tapes. Wrap one anchor tape around the middle of the thigh (k) and the other around the base of your calf (l). Your kneecap will remain exposed.

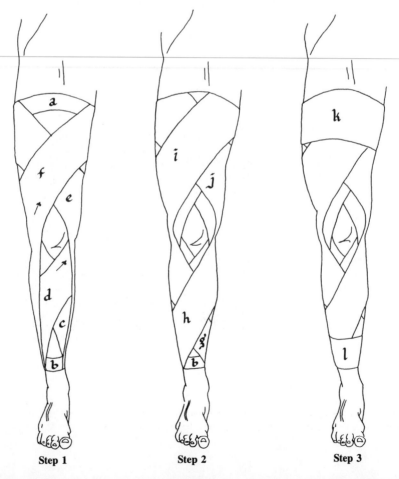

Step 1   Step 2   Step 3

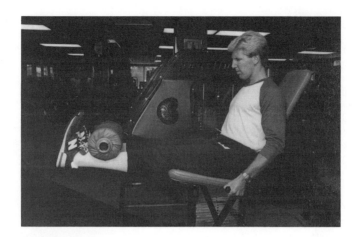

Sprained Knee

Rehabilitative Exercise #1

For this exercise, use the Nautilus Leg Extension machine or some other form of resistance. Sit down and slowly extend your right leg until it is straight. Hold this position for 1 second and then repeat the exercise for 2 sets of 15 reps. Increase the weight as you build up your tolerance.

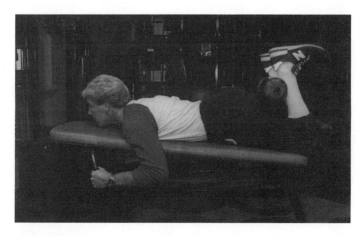

Sprained Knee

Rehabilitative Exercise #2

For this exercise, use the Nautilus Leg Curl machine or some other form of resistance. Lie on your stomach and slowly curl your right heel toward your right buttock. Hold this position for 1 second and then repeat the exercise for 2 sets of 15 reps. Increase the weight as you build up your tolerance.

Sprained Knee

Rehabilitative Exercise #3
Increase the endurance of your quadriceps and hamstrings through swimming or using a stationary bicycle. Both are excellent forms of exercise. Begin with 5 minutes of exercise and lengthen the duration as you build up your tolerance.

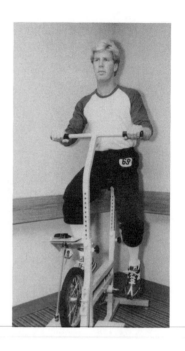

Sprained Wrist

Symptoms: Tenderness and restricted mobility of the wrist.

Causes: Forcing the wrist into a position beyond its extended range of motion, such as falling onto your outstreched hand while fielding a baseball.

Protective Support: Support the affected area with wrist taping.

Sprained Wrist

Wrist Taping
Materials: One roll of 1-inch adhesive tape.

Position of Player: Hold your injured wrist in a relaxed fashion. Spread your fingers as wide as possible.

Procedure: As shown in Step #1, wrap a strip of 1-inch adhesive tape around your wrist just above the base of the thumb and just below the wrist bone (a).

As shown in Step #2, wrap three more strips progressively higher up the lower forearm (b,c,d). Each strip of tape should overlap half of the preceding strip.

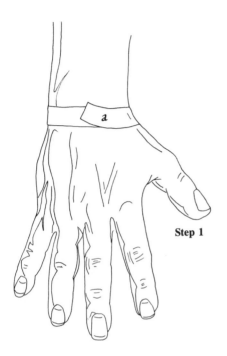

Step 1

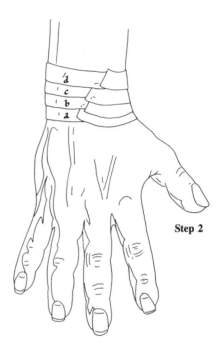

Step 2

Sprained Wrist

Rehabilitative Exercise #1

Sit in a chair. Bend your knees and place your feet flat on the floor. Place your right forearm on your right thigh. Your wrist should hang over your knee. Bend your elbow at a 90° angle and position your hand "palm up." Make a fist and slowly pull your right hand upward. Hold this position for 1 second and then repeat the exercise for 2 sets of 15 reps. Begin this exercise using no weight. You may add weight, however, as you build up your tolerance.

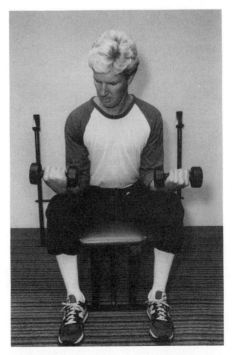

Sprained Wrist

Rehabilitative Exercise #2

Sit in a chair. Bend your knees and place your feet flat on the floor. Place your right forearm on your right thigh. Your wrist should hang over your knee. Bend your elbow at a 90°angle and position your hand "palm down." Make a fist and slowly pull your right hand upward. Hold this position for 1 second and then repeat the exercise for 2 sets of 15 reps. Begin this exercise using no weight. You may add weight, however, as you build up your tolerance.

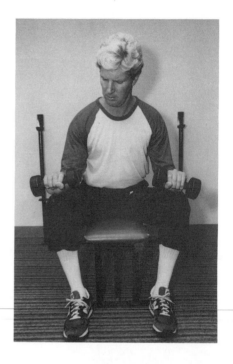

Sprained Wrist

Rehabilitative Exercise #3

Sit in a chair. Bend your knees and place your feet flat on the floor. Place your right forearm on your right thigh. Your wrist should hang over your knee. Bend your elbow at a 90°angle. Begin the exercise with your right hand in a "palm up" position. Using a dumbbell with the weight on one end of the bar only, slowly rotate your right hand counterclockwise until your hand is in a "palm down" position. Hold this position for 1 second, then repeat the exercise for 2 sets of 15 reps. Use a light weight initially and increase the weight as you build up your tolerance. The exercise also can be made more challenging by grasping the dumbbell farther away from the weights.

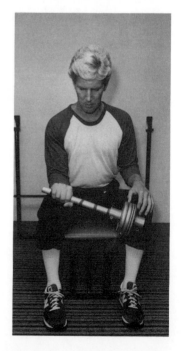

Sprained Wrist

Rehabilitative Exercise #4

Grasp a rubber ball or a PRO "Sports Grip" with your right hand. Squeeze the ball or grip and concentrate on contracting your forearm muscles. Hold the contraction for 1 second, then repeat the exercise 30 times.

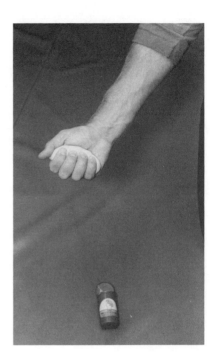

Chapter

8

The Ballpark Diet

Next to the players themselves, the most appreciated people at a baseball game are the food vendors. There's something about baseball games that drives people to eat. Hot dogs, popcorn, beer, and soda are all time-honored, traditional fare that true baseball fans love to munch.

As popular as they are, however, foods like these are poor dietary choices for spectators, let alone baseball players. They may taste great, especially amid the heat, dust, and excitement of competition. But they are filled with empty calories and are nutritionally unsound. Unfortunately, too many athletes fill their diets with foods as devoid of nutritional value as the ballpark diets of their fans. They may keep their bodies in super shape otherwise, but they neglect to include sensible eating habits as part of their overall conditioning routine. Ignoring their bodies' nutritional needs impairs their performances on the field.

Because wise eating is so important to athletes' health, many sports medicine centers include nutritional counseling as a part of their prevention and treatment programs. Counselors evaluate players' eating habits and recommend dietary changes designed to satisfy each athlete's nutritional and caloric requirements. Sports nutritionists develop diets not only for preseason and in-season activites but also for year-round dietary needs. Like exercise, the experts say, balanced meals must be a lifelong habit, not just something you are forced to do while you are active in sports.

What to Eat

Nutrition awareness has grown so much during the past decade that athletes no longer have difficulties learning what foods are best to meet their bodies' dietary needs. But if you have never obtained information regarding sensible nutrition, use this chapter as a primer for the more comprehensive nutrition information sources available. Many good books and articles on the subject are in print that are very worthwhile to read.

Simply put, your body requires 40 fundamental nutrients to function properly. These nutrients can be divided into seven categories: water, carbohydrates, protein, fat, electrolytes, vitamins, and minerals.

All the nutrients you need can be easily obtained by eating balanced meals. Few sports nutritionists recommend supplementary aids or salt tablets because the athletes who watch their diets are seldom nutrient-deficient, although the addition of a daily multiple vitamin/mineral is an effective safeguard. Health conscious players satisfy their nutritional needs by eating several servings daily of the following four food groups:

Milk: Two or more servings
Meat: Two or more servings (depending upon injury status)
Fruits and vegetables: Four or more servings (depending upon caloric needs)
Grains: Four or more servings (depending upon caloric needs)

Three nutrient categories—carbohydrates, proteins, and fats—provide your muscles with the fuel you need for peak performance during competition.

Carbohydrates (60-65% of Diet)
Of the three types of fuel nutrients, carbohydrates are the best source of energy, especially for muscles that are exercised strenuously. Stored in the muscles and liver as muscle sugar (glycogen), carbohydrates are digested more quickly and easily than proteins and fats and are thus readily available when you need them for energy. Thus carbohydrates are a great precompetition food.

Carbohydrates can be found in junk foods such as candy or soda and in foods rich in starch, such as pasta, potatoes, bread, rice, cereals, and vegetables. Although both food types provide you with fuel, obtain your carbohydrates from starches (complex carbohydrates) rather than from sweets. This approach will enable you to meet your carbohydrate needs without risking the sugar highs and lows that can lead to severe health disorders.

Proteins (15-20% of Diet)
Proteins are also an energy source but are used by your body primarily to build tissues. Proteins are vital nutrients but cannot be digested as easily as carbohydrates. Many athletes believe that meats, which are high in fat, and eggs, which are high in cholesterol, are their best sources of protein, but this is not true. All the protein you need can be acquired through small portions of poultry, fish, yogurt, and milk.

Fats (20-25% of Diet)
Fats are the most concentrated form of energy. Fats insulate your body, protect it from injury, and help to hold your organs in position. Athletes need fat, but they don't need it in the quantities that most players consume. Excess fat is exactly that—fat. The fat you do not burn builds up in your body, something like an unwanted party guest.

Like proteins, fats are much harder to digest than carbohydrates. So eat fatty foods only in moderation. Beef, butter, pork, cream, and fried foods may taste great, but they are not especially beneficial to your athletic performance and can be harmful if not consumed in moderation.

What to Drink

Water is the best fluid for your body. All those fancy "drinks" designed especially for athletes can't hold a candle to the benefits of water. Water is easily absorbed and replenishes body fluids lost through perspiration more quickly than other liquids. Juices and other drinks may provide you with necessary electrolytes (sodium, potassium, and chloride), but your body still loves most what it's made of most—water. The professional athletes drink water before, during, and after games and practices.

When to Eat

Daily Eating Pattern
There's nothing wrong with eating three balanced meals a day, but there's also nothing wrong with eating more than three times daily. Intelligent snacking is an excellent means of maintaining high energy and stamina levels. As long as your caloric intake remains the same, you will not gain weight regardless of how frequently you eat. In fact, many athletes find that smaller, more frequent meals help them to lose weight. Faced with fewer hours of hunger between meals, they no longer view breakfast, lunch, and dinner as "gorge time."

Eating Before Exercise
There's a reason that your parents told you not to swim right after you eat, and that reason applies to any form of exercise, not only swimming. As you exercise, the muscles you work the hardest require the most fuel, which is oxygen. Muscles receive oxygen from your bloodstream, which diverts blood from less demanding parts of your body to satisfy the oxygen needs of the muscles being exercised. One area that suffers reduced blood flow during exercise is the stomach. Because your stomach muscles require oxygen to digest food, you should avoid eating for 3 hours before you exercise. If you eat during that period, much of the food may not be digested by the

time you exercise. Faced with food to be digested and a reduced oxygen supply, your stomach muscles will become anoxic (without oxygen) and will rebel by cramping. Doubled over with pain, you'll stop exercising. The bloodstream will redivert blood to your complaining stomach muscles until their oxygen demands are satisfied and your food has been digested. Then you'll be able to exercise again, but the discomfort and strain you have experienced may lead you to halt your workout altogether.

You can avoid these problems as well as the onset of fatigue associated with a hypoglycemic response when you eat no longer than 5 hours before exercise and no sooner than 3 hours.

Eating During Exercise
Most players do not eat while they are exercising or competing. They're just too busy, and eating doesn't occur to them. Besides, eating puts food into the stomach and can cause real discomfort.

If you get hungry, however, while you're sitting in the dugout, eat lightly and eat easily digested carbohydrates. Fruits are good choices. Better yet, drink a fluid replacement energy drink such as EXCEED. It not only will satisfy your hunger but will also help to replenish the liquids, carbohydrates, and electrolytes lost during exercise and reduce the danger of dehydration and fatigue.

How Much to Eat

Athletes burn more calories when they are active than when they are inactive. This is true for all people. People's caloric needs change as they expend varying amounts of energy.

Most athletes require 3,000–6,000 calories daily during preseason training and in-season competition. That caloric intake will satisfy the body's energy demands as it performs. As a baseball player, you may spend part of any game standing inactive in the field or sitting on the bench. Thus your caloric needs may be less than those of a runner or soccer player. But if you exercise vigorously and regularly to prepare for competition, you will still require far more calories a day than the average person.

During the off season, regulate your caloric intake according to the amount of exercise you continue to do. If you work out regularly, your caloric intake will remain similar to that of preseason and in-season activity. If you neglect your conditioning program, make certain that you reduce the number of calories you eat. Otherwise you will gain weight or even become fat, and it will be that much harder to get back into shape when preseason training resumes.

Whatever your caloric needs, be sure to satisfy the demand through sensible, nutritious eating. Don't fill yourself with empty calories. Instead, eat more of the good foods found in any balanced diet.

Fluid demands also increase when you are active. As you perspire, you lose water, which must be replaced to avoid dehydration. The more you exercise, the more fluids you should drink. There's no danger of drinking too much fluid because your body will eliminate any excess through urination. Dehydration can result in muscle impairment, fatigue, and in extreme cases even death. So saturate your tissues with the fluids they need.

Index

About the Author

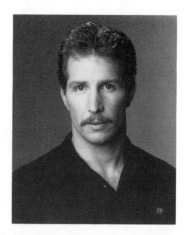

Pat Croce is president of Sports Physical Therapists, Inc., and is currently on staff at Holy Redeemer Hospital in Huntington Valley, PA. A licensed physical therapist and a certified athletic trainer, he also serves as physical conditioning coach for the Philadelphia Flyers and physical therapist for both the Philadelphia 76'ers and members of the Philadelphia Phillies.

A native of Philadelphia, Pat Croce is a graduate of the University of Pittsburgh. He is an elected member of both the American College of Sports Medicine and the National Strength and Conditioning Association. He is active in both broadcasting and journalism, hosting "The Pat Croce Show" daily on WIP Radio (610AM) and co-hosting "Fit In" on WCAU-TV (CBS), as well as writing the "Personal Fitness" feature for the Philadelphia Sunday *Inquirer*. He has authored three books on the fields of fitness and sports medicine, and has written for such national magazines as *Sports Fitness, Superfit, Drug Therapy, Feeling Great, Bicycling,* and *Goal Magazine*.

Pat Croce currently resides in Bryn Mawr, PA, with his wife Diane and his two children, Kelly and Michael. In his leisure time Pat enjoys competing in a variety of activities, and has won the United States National Karate Championship twice.